For Lou D'Angelo —
another addition to
your NAG bibliography,
with the admiration
and affection of the author —

Neil A. Grauer

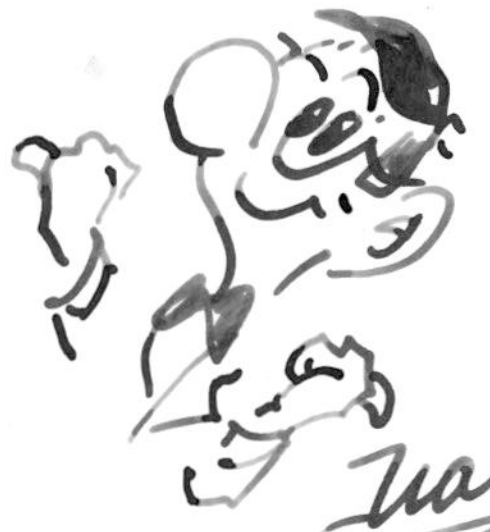

THE FULL
SIGNATURE
WILL MAKE IT
MORE VALUABLE
ON E-BAY...!

NAG

Baltimore,
July 16, 2004

*Dedicated to the physicians, nurses, residents, interns,
employees, volunteers, trustees—and patients—of the
Johns Hopkins Bayview Medical Center,
past, present and future.*

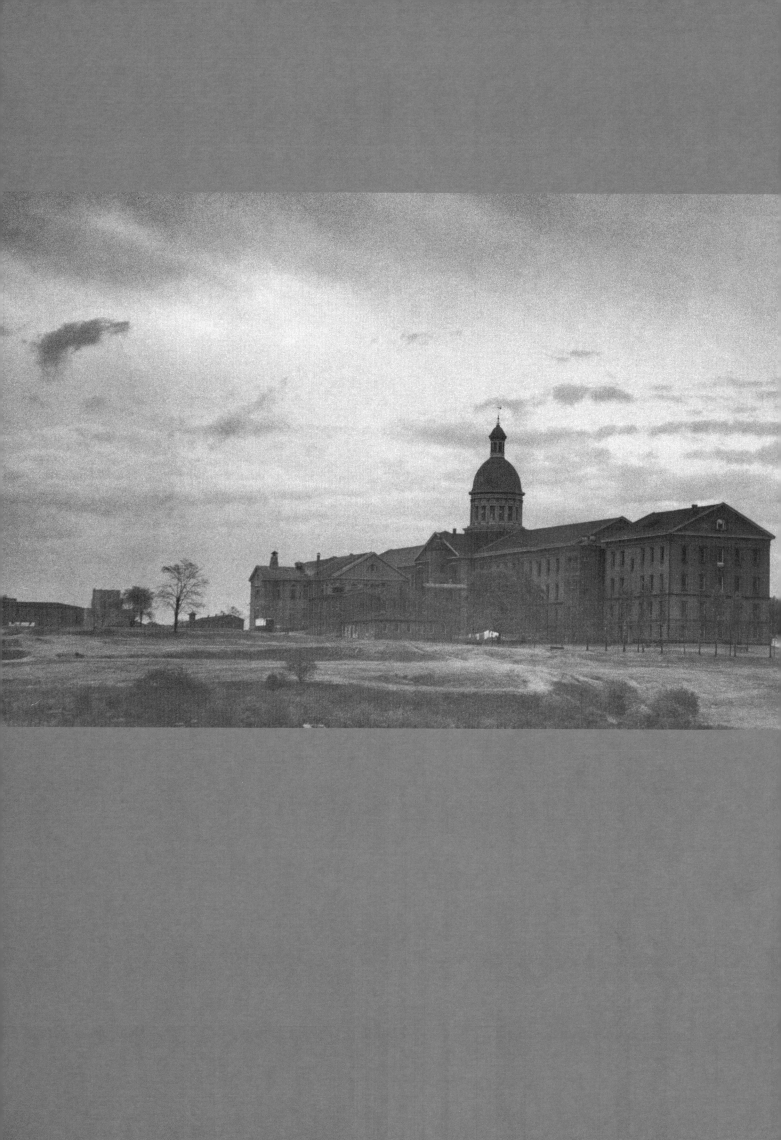

CENTURIES OF CARING

The Johns Hopkins Bayview Medical Center Story

by Neil A. Grauer
Johns Hopkins 2004

This book has been brought to publication with the generous support
of the Trustees of the Johns Hopkins Bayview Medical Center.

Copyright © 2004 by The Johns Hopkins University and Johns Hopkins Health System
All rights reserved.

Published and distributed by the Johns Hopkins Medicine Health Publishing Business
Group, Office of Corporate Communications, Johns Hopkins Medicine
901 S. Bond Street, Suite 550
Baltimore, MD 21231

ISBN 0-9755326-1-8

Library of Congress Control Number: 2004107002

Vice President, Corporate Communications: Elaine Freeman
Production Coordinator: Steve Libowitz
Copy Editor: Eileen O'Brien
Design Direction: Max Boam, Johns Hopkins Medicine Office of Corporate Communications
Designer: Peter Owen
Photographers: Mike Ciesielski, Bill Klosicki, David Kurniawan, Milton Tudahl,
Kevin Weber, Keith Weller and Richard Yienger
Printed in the United States by PMR Printing Company

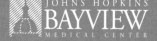

Previous spread: Dawn breaks over City Hospitals' landmark
1866 asylum—now the Mason F. Lord Building—on New
Year's Day, 1951. (Photo by Albert D. Cochran, ©1951 *The
Baltimore Sun.* Used by permission.)

Contents

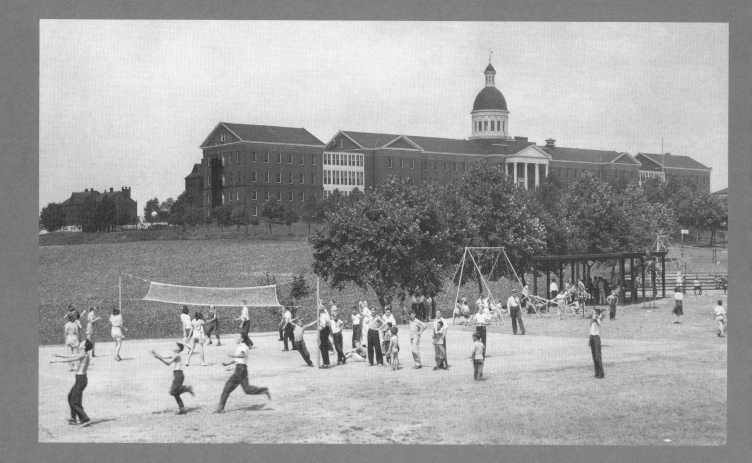

Highlandtown youngsters enjoy themselves on the City Hospitals' playground in August 1939. (©1939 *The Baltimore Sun.* Used by permission.)

Acknowledgements

ALTHOUGH AN AUTHOR ALONE PUTS PEN TO paper (or fingers to word processor), no history such as this could be written without the cooperation, advice and support of many individuals.

Ronald R. Peterson, president of The Johns Hopkins Hospital and Johns Hopkins Health System, provided the initial support, encouragement and advice for this project. As the former president of the Johns Hopkins Bayview Medical Center, he has a unique, comprehensive knowledge of its fascinating history—as well as a deep awareness of how worthwhile telling its story would be. Mr. Peterson's successor as president of Hopkins Bayview, Gregory Schaffer, has been equally supportive and helpful.

Physicians are the soul of any hospital. Hopkins Bayview has been blessed by the dedicated medical care and devotion of outstanding practitioners for most of its history, and never more so than over the past half-century. Those physicians who gave generously of their insights and recollections for the writing of this book include Philip Zieve, Chester Schmidt Jr., Burton D'Lugoff, John R. Burton, L. Reuven Pasternak, David Spector and Robert Spence.

The administrators and trustees, past and present, who worked so closely with the medical staff at Hopkins Bayview to ensure its survival and expansion were just as helpful to this author. They include Judy Reitz, L. Kenneth Grabill II, William Ward, Robert D. H. Harvey, William McCarthy, Francis Knott, Edward Halle and Walter Sondheim Jr.

At Hopkins Bayview, few have a finer understanding of the community it serves than Gayle Johnson Adams, director of community and government relations; P. Susan Davis, director of communications and public affairs; and Sandy Reckert, editor of *Bayview News,* and its designer, Cynthia Herrick, all of whom provided invaluable assistance. Crucial help also was given by Linda Gorman, director of Hopkins Bayview's library services; her associates, Irene Kiyatkin and Tillie Horak; and in the Office of Media Services, by Dave Kurniawan, Keishia Pratt and Bill Klosicki, a mainstay of the hospital's media services department since before "media" was a commonly employed word.

Significant aid also was rendered by Nancy McCall and Andrew Harrison of Hopkins's Alan Mason Chesney Medical Archives; the staff of the Enoch Pratt Free Library; the Welch Medical Library; Maryland Historical Society; MedChi, the Maryland State Medical Society; the Baltimore Museum of Art; the Hearst Corporation, and the University of Maryland's Hornbake Library, repository of the Baltimore *News American* photograph collection; *The Baltimore Sun* and the Tribune Company; and the Maryland State Police.

Help—and indulgence—also were abundant from those at my base of operations, the Office of Corporate Communications of Johns Hopkins Medicine. Director Elaine Freeman; deputy director Joann Rodgers; publications director Edith Nichols; associate director of publications Patrick Gilbert; designers Peter Owen and Maxwell J. Boam; Steve Libowitz, director of the Health Publishing Business Group, and copy editor Eileen O'Brien were instrumental in ensuring that this book not only was published—but done so handsomely.

Neil A. Grauer
Baltimore
July 1, 2004

INTRODUCTIONS

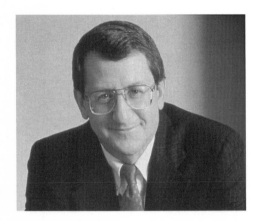

AS WE CELEBRATE THE 20TH ANNIVERSARY OF THE ACQUISITION of the former Baltimore City Hospitals by The Johns Hopkins Hospital and University, those of us who had the privilege of serving the Bayview organization during that time are pleased to recall witnessing the remarkable transformation of a proud public hospital system.

This was accomplished during an era when many similar institutions around the country failed to work successfully through the privatization process. As Mr. Grauer has so ably reminded us in his marvelous recounting of Hopkins Bayview's unique story, several important ingredients combined to create a successful recipe for revitalization. The well-organized and committed clinical practice organization of Hopkins faculty on the scene managed to work as partners with a band of Hopkins administrators dispatched by the visionary Dr. Robert Heyssel. The partnership of faculty and administrative leaders, in tandem with a dedicated board of trustees assigned by Johns Hopkins, built upon the unique programmatic opportunities available on this very special campus. In addition, with the passage of time, as Dr. Philip Zieve importantly observes, the organization continuously adapted in a constructive manner to environmental challenges.

The recent merger of the faculty practices at Hopkins Bayview and Hopkins Hospital will enable an ever-wiser approach in the future to joint program planning across the Hopkins campuses. Bayview will become an increasingly important contributor to Johns Hopkins Medicine's tripartite mission of research, teaching and patient care—without becoming a clone of The Johns Hopkins Hospital.

No matter what the future may portend in terms of corporate structural changes, it is my belief that Bayview will continue to maintain its own culture. As such, Bayview will carry on its long-standing tradition of serving the citizens of Southeast Baltimore and beyond with the best possible contemporary health care services as a proud member of Johns Hopkins Medicine.

Ronald R. Peterson
President, The Johns Hopkins Hospital
President, Johns Hopkins Health System

BASED ON WHAT MY FATHER HAD TOLD ME OF THE OLD BALTIMORE City Hospitals, I was amazed when I first visited the campus of the Johns Hopkins Bayview Medical Center in 1995. Instead of the often-grim municipal institution recalled by my dad, a student in Baltimore from the late 1920s to the mid-1930s, I found a campus that had undergone an astounding transformation.

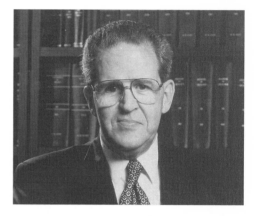

Old buildings had come down or been completely rebuilt inside; new buildings had gone up; the atmosphere was one of enormous progress, not of a painstaking attempt to remain afloat amid overwhelming odds.

Today I continue to be amazed by the vitality and promise of this extraordinary hospital—and excited about meeting the challenges we face to maintain and advance those remarkable achievements in the years ahead.

In the two decades since we became a member of the Johns Hopkins family, Hopkins Bayview has seen patient admissions nearly double to more than 20,000 a year and outpatient visits double to some 150,000 annually. We also have expanded our research activities immensely. Clearly we need more space for these critically important endeavors.

Throughout Hopkins Bayview's 230 years of history, change has been a constant—as has been the commitment to serve our community to the best of our ability. The closer collaboration of Hopkins Bayview and The Johns Hopkins Hospital, facilitated by the merger of our two School of Medicine clinical practices, is certain to ensure that we will meet the challenges ahead with even greater vigor.

As we become more closely aligned with Hopkins Hospital, we also must remain true to our own traditions, which are so ably instilled by our employees on each generation of their successors. This hospital has a wonderful personality—part of which remains from its days as City Hospitals. When it often was the hospital of last resort for this region's poor, it attracted employees whose care for patients was rendered with genuine compassion. That has stayed with us—and I think it will be here for a long time to come.

Gregory F. Schaffer

Gregory F. Schaffer
President, Johns Hopkins Bayview Medical Center

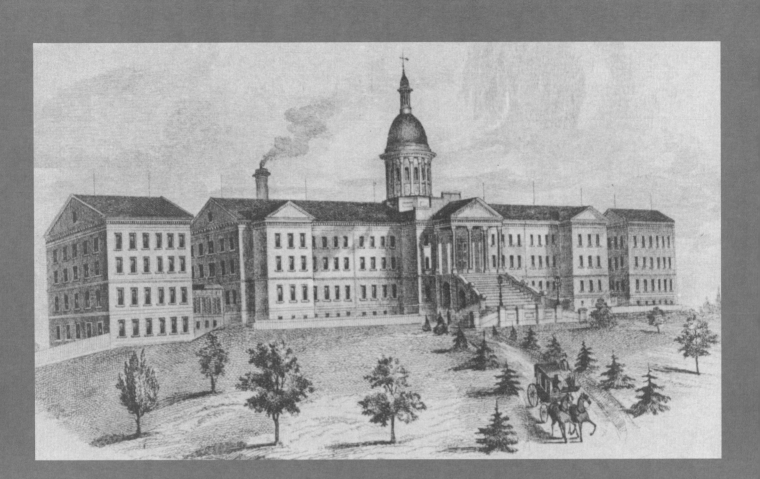

A mid-19th century engraving of the original three-story main building of the Bay View Almshouse, erected in 1866 on a hill overlooking the Chesapeake Bay. Repeatedly renovated, then completely gutted and expanded to five floors, it now is known as the Mason F. Lord Building. Its dome was removed in 1954 after city engineers judged it to be unstable, though it proved difficult to dismantle. (Hopkins Bayview Biomedical Media Services [HBBMS])

1

"For the reception and lodging of the poor . . . [and] a Doctor for his salary and medicines"

BALTIMORE IN 1773 MAY HAVE CALLED ITSELF A CITY, BUT IN REALITY it was a small town of fewer than 6,000 souls that aspired to become a major metropolis. Its unpaved streets turned to mud in the rain and were unlit at night. (The local newspaper called for the installation of streetlights so people would not stumble into a "quagmire" in the dark.) Most of the structures in the city were wooden, although there was a stone courthouse and a number of brick merchants' houses. Inns, a theater, a town marketplace and a harbor filled with commercial vessels attested to Baltimore's potential for growth.[1]

As the nascent city advanced, its urban ills expanded; all increased the numbers of indigent infirm or sick people, petty criminals, vagrants and beggars. In 1773, the Maryland legislature authorized the purchase of 20 acres for an Almshouse "for the reception and lodging of the poor," as well as to pay for "a Doctor . . . and his medicines." The Almshouse was to be located on a site bounded by present-day Linden Avenue and Eutaw, Biddle and Madison streets, then outside the northwest border of the city in what was Baltimore County. The price of the property was 350 pounds of tobacco, then a common currency.[2]

The land was graded, two 70-foot wells were dug, the Almshouse buildings were erected and the property landscaped.[3] In 1774, the Baltimore City and County Almshouse—the first institutional ancestor of the Baltimore City Hospitals and ultimately the Johns Hopkins Bayview Medical Center—opened its doors.[4]

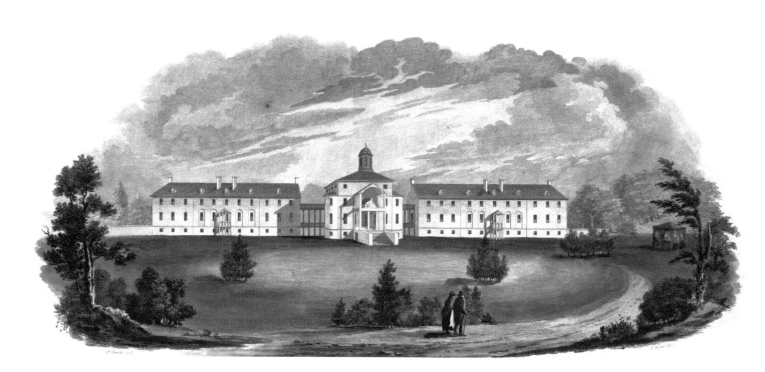

The Almshouse at Calverton, 1824. Converted from the former estate of a bankrupt Baltimore businessman, it sometimes was derided as "The Paupers' Palace." Built on reclaimed swampland, it was an unhealthy location for treating the sick. (Maryland Historical Society)

Almshouses in the 18th century were not hospitals as we know them today but places that offered temporary shelter for the homeless, defendants awaiting trial or convicted criminals, who were required to work for their keep. These institutions functioned simultaneously as infirmaries that provided rudimentary care for foundlings, the insane and the impoverished sick, infirm or elderly. Early almshouse infirmaries often became hospitals, including Philadelphia General Hospital, founded as an almshouse in 1729 (closed in 1977); New York's Bellevue Hospital, founded as an almshouse in 1731; and New Orleans' Charity Hospital, founded in 1732.[5]

The domed central building of the Baltimore Almshouse was flanked by east and west wings. It had two sections: a Workhouse, where beggars, vagrants and petty criminals had to work; and an Almshouse, where, from the outset, a visiting physician would care for the ill residents in its infirmary.[6]

The original Almshouse was heavily damaged by fire in September 1776. The main building promptly was rebuilt, but the damaged east wing took longer to repair. No records exist from this time describing the Almshouse's appearance, the number of beds provided for the sick, or the number of people who lived there, but annual reports suggest they led a spare existence. Every resident had a small, whitewashed room that was sanitized each fall and spring with boiling water and quicklime. Every adult had a bed with a straw-filled cotton mattress and a blanket that was laundered twice a year. Children were kept two to a bed.[7]

Baltimore emerged from the American Revolution a far more important city. In 1777, as British troops threatened Philadelphia, Congress reconvened in Baltimore, briefly making it the nation's capital. War trade expanded the city's role as a commercial center, and its population grew to 8,000 by the war's end, still behind that of Boston, New York or Philadelphia, but nonetheless substantial. By 1790, Baltimore had become the fastest-growing city in the young United States, with a population of 13,500. By 1800, Baltimore's size had nearly doubled to 26,514, supplanting Boston (with 24,937 residents) as the country's third-largest city after New York (60,515) and Philadelphia (41,220).[8] There was ample need for the Almshouse's services.

Douglas G. Carroll Jr., (1915-1977) was chief of physical medicine and rehabilitation at Baltimore City Hospitals, a descendant of Revolutionary-era patriot Charles Carroll the Barrister, and a scholar of the institution's history. He noted in a series of articles published by the Maryland State Medical Journal in 1966, that physicians in late 18th century America could be grouped into three categories. A few had been well trained in Europe under the tutelage of highly respected doctors; others served as apprentices to practicing physicians in this country, reading medical textbooks and often serving as their mentors' pharmacist to learn about the compounding of medications. Still others served brief medical apprenticeships, took some lecture courses offered by what passed for American medical schools, and with this scant training (no license was required) proclaimed themselves physicians. Many were quacks, of course, but even the best-educated doctors had little knowledge about diagnosing most internal illnesses. Only readily discernable afflictions and major external injuries were immediately recognized and treated.[9]

The Baltimore Almshouse was fortunate to have a number of distinguished doctors serve as visiting physicians. In 1789, Andrew Wiesenthal (1762-1798), the son of a prominent city doctor, was appointed attending physician shortly after he returned to Baltimore following three years of study at St. Bartholomew's Hospital in London. Wiesenthal, a talented diagnostician, achieved a significant medical breakthrough when he determined that a roundworm in the trachea of domestic fowl was the cause of syngmosis ("the gapes"), an important epizootic disease. This was the first discovery of the link between an organism and an infectious disease or epidemic.[10]

Wiesenthal even endeavored to found a medical school in Baltimore, offering lectures on anatomy and surgery in 1789-90 to a class of 15 students. Another well-trained doctor, George Buchanan, gave lectures on diseases common to women and children. This experiment in medical education ended when Wiesenthal died in 1798 at the tragically young age of 36.

Following Wiesenthal as resident physician at the Baltimore Almshouse was James Smith (1771-1841), a student of the renowned Benjamin Rush at the University of Pennsylvania. Smith served from 1800 to 1801 and became

The original Baltimore City and County Almshouse of 1774-1822. This is the only known depiction of the first Baltimore Almshouse. It appears on an 1801 map of Baltimore. (HBBMS)

N.os Admission	Dates of Admission	Names	Ages Yrs mnths	By whom Admitted	How, when & by whom Discharged	Remarks
2021	Sept 7 1818	Hannah Myers	60	R Waters	April 1 1819 imployd as Cook	June 10. 1820. Disc being Cook — for g drunk repeatedly
2022	Octr 27	Elizabeth Robinson	19	Jn McPhirson	Novbr 2 1818 By J M & their Request	Sore Nee ___ taken away by Mrs Niss
2023	— 28	Eleazer Henery		R Waters	March 5 1819 By Death	Blind
2024	— 28	Michel Bryan		Jn Ellicott	Novbr 21 1818 By J M & his Request	Scurvey by Towid
2025	—	J. George Shenaman	55	J W G	Apl. 13. 1819 By Job Merryman	Stiff neck
2026	— 29	Elishea Dorsey		J W G	Octor 22 1818 By J M & his Request	fits
2027	—	Daniel Madden		J W G	May 24 1819 By J M & his Request	Blind
		Christian	30	Jn Ellicott	April 6 1819	

Baltimore Almshouse Admission Book page from September 1818 lists such reasons for patient admission as "blind" and "stiff neck." Other entries from the period list admission causes as "deranged," "a drunken fellow," "consumption" and "poverty." (HBBMS)

known as the father of vaccination in Maryland when he inoculated 7-year-old Almshouse resident Nancy Malcum against smallpox on May 1, 1801. This was Maryland's first vaccination. It came just three years after England's Edward Jenner published his findings that vaccination with the less dangerous cow pox could prevent the spread of smallpox and less than a year after Harvard professor Benjamin Waterhouse performed the first vaccination in the United States in Cambridge, Massachusetts, inoculating his own 5-year-old son and others against smallpox on July 8, 1800.[11]

Smith became a powerful advocate of vaccination in the United States, garnering sufficient prominence that his portrait was painted by Rembrandt Peale, the foremost portraitist of the day, and earning him praise in *The Med-*

ical Annals of Maryland, which called him "the Jenner of America."[12]

Neither Wiesenthal nor Smith had used Almshouse residents as subjects for medical instruction. When William Gibson and Samuel Baker, both professors of surgery at the College of Medicine of Maryland (later the University of Maryland Medical School), accepted appointments as visiting physicians around 1812, however, they insisted that their students be given access to Almshouse patients for medical training. This consisted primarily of surgical procedures undertaken without the benefit of anesthesia, which did not come into use until the 1840s.

According to an Almshouse admission and discharge book, there were approximately 8,317 admissions from 1814 to 1826. Some were criminals, sentenced to serve up to seven years in the Workhouse. Some were foundlings. Other reasons listed for admission were "blind," "deranged," "idiotism," "a drunken fellow," "a vagrant," "consumption," "pregnant," and, quite simply, "poverty."[13] Most residents remained for only a few months; some stayed for years. One patient admitted in 1778 still was there in 1814.

By 1818, the trustees of the Almshouse could report to the city government that its staff included a full-time physician, seven visiting doctors and surgeons, a druggist and a matron.[14] Would-be physicians continued to use the Almshouse as a medical teaching facility. Two medical students paid $150 each to live there for two years, and other students of medicine and surgery were encouraged to join the visiting physicians on their rounds—for a fee of $10.

Increasingly, the Almshouse concentrated on treating the sick as other organizations started to take charge of the orphans, the criminals and the insane previously housed there. The Baltimore Female Orphan Society was founded in 1808 to provide care and schooling to impoverished orphans. In 1811, the newly built Maryland Penitentiary in Baltimore became the place to send criminals who did not belong in the Workhouse. In 1828, the state began placing some of the indigent insane in the Maryland Hospital, which stood on the East Baltimore site now occupied by The Johns Hopkins Hospital and soon confined its role to that of an insane asylum. As the Almshouse assumed a

James Smith (1771-1841), a student of Benjamin Rush at the University of Pennsylvania (1794) and resident physician at the Baltimore City and County Almshouse (1800-01). He performed Maryland's first vaccination against smallpox at the Almshouse on May 1, 1801. His efforts to promote vaccination in the United States earned him the sobriquet "the Jenner of America." This portrait was painted between 1813 and 1815 by Rembrandt Peale (1778-1860), the most prominent portraitist of the time. (The Baltimore Museum of Art)

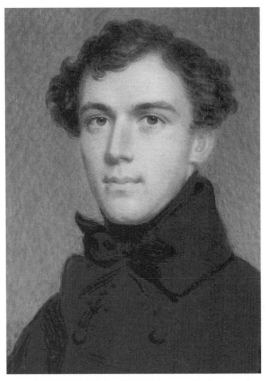

William Power (1813-1852), resident physician, Baltimore Almshouse (1840). He introduced scientific medicine to Baltimore, taking careful medical histories of Almshouse patients. (Med-Chi, The Maryland State Medical Society)

more focused medical role, Baltimore's top doctors readily offered their services to provide care and teach medicine there. Prominent physicians and citizens willingly accepted appointment to its board of trustees.[15]

As Baltimore began outgrowing its original boundaries, the land on which the Almshouse stood became prime property for prospective residences. To make way for them, in 1819 the city and county spent $44,000 to purchase Calverton, the 306-acre estate of Dennis A. Smith, a city merchant who had lost much of his fortune in a financial panic that year. His classical-style stone mansion sat atop a hill surrounded, "in the English style," with walls, gardens, meadows, stands of elm and willow trees and an apple orchard. The property, located in a rural area now bordered by Franklin, Presstman, Lexington and Pulaski streets in West Baltimore, contained separate bath and wash houses, a bakery, a spinning house—even a morgue. As a result of Smith's shaky finances, it all became the property of the Mechanics' Bank, which sold Calverton to the city as a replacement for the Almshouse. Once all 533 Almshouse residents were moved there in December 1822, it inevitably became known as the "paupers' palace." Beginning in 1823, new patients were admitted for health care.[16]

The mansion's apparently lush surroundings obscured the swampland on which it was built. Accommodations were far from luxurious for the residents. Paupers were housed in the basement; sick and old people were put in windowed rooms upstairs. In 1826, the trustees reported the annual cost of housing a poor person was $37.63. Within a few years, they had reduced that expense by almost one-third to just $25.72. The trustees made certain that all beggars and vagabonds sent to Calverton worked for their keep at carpentry, maintenance, dairy farming and tending the huge vegetable garden that provided much of the residents' food.[17] The fare evidently was sufficient but monotonous: breakfast and lunch both were bread and molasses, accompanied by coffee or tea with sugar. Dinners followed a regular pattern: mutton and soup on Mondays and Thursdays; mush or rice with molasses or hominy on Tuesdays and Fridays; beef and soup on Wednesdays and Saturdays; pork or bacon with vegetables on Sundays.[18]

The Calverton mansion was expanded to nearly a city block in length by the addition of two institutional-style wings. No establishment in America administering to "the wants of the wretched" appeared more impressive, wrote a foreign observer in 1830.[19] Calverton may have looked splendid, but it turned out to be a hellish place for a health facility. Its water supply was vulnerable to raw sewage, and its swampy acreage was a fertile breeding ground for disease-carrying mosquitoes.[20]

The Almshouse at Calverton retained the multiple responsibilities of its predecessor. It cared for the impoverished ill, served as a lying-in hospital for poor women, maintained a workhouse for vagrants, took in penniless children, housed the insane and acted as a school for medicine and surgery. "One can well imagine the bedlam," Carroll wrote in the mid-20th century.[21] Yet Carroll also saw signs of "modern" treatment philosophy even in that inhospitable setting. The diagnoses of mental patients included "disappointed affection," "indulgence of passion and pride" and "religious perplexity," suggesting that "humane, sophisticated" concepts of mental illness were emerging, however slowly.[22]

A surge of sick immigrants in 1831 put added strain on the facility. A cholera outbreak in 1832 claimed 125 patients out of approximately 500 in residence. In 1849, cholera ravaged both the city and Calverton, killing 94 of the 158 individuals treated there. The causes of cholera were unknown then, and treatment was primitive. In fact, physicians then had no laboratory tests to distinguish malaria from typhoid, or typhus from dysentery or tuberculosis. Infants at Calverton were especially susceptible to fatal illnesses—cholera in the summer, pneumonia in the winter. "In the whole history of the establishment, there is no single example of a foundling that lived to the age of three years," wrote Thomas H. Buckler in 1851.[23]

Despite this dismal record, it was at the Calverton Almshouse that William Power (1813-1852) inaugurated the practice of scientific medicine in Baltimore when he became resident physician there in 1840. A Baltimore native, an 1831 graduate of Yale and a medical student at the Almshouse in 1834, the year before he graduated from the University of Maryland School of Medicine, Power "introduced careful medical history, the new methods of percussion and auscultation in the physical examination, proper progress notes, and careful postmortem examination to try to understand the nature of disease," Carroll wrote.[24] Because of Power's

Bay View Asylum Certificate, 1874. The name of the Almshouse was changed to Asylum to reflect its role as an insane asylum, as well as its other medical and societal functions. **(HBBMS)**

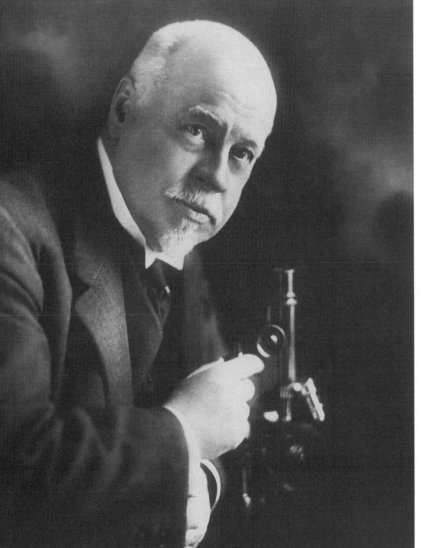

William Welch (1850-1934), the first professor of pathology at the Johns Hopkins School of Medicine. He established the first connection between Hopkins and the Bay View Asylum as a venue for teaching medical students in 1885. (The Alan Mason Chesney Medical Archives of The Johns Hopkins Medical Institutions)

innovations, residents of the Baltimore Almshouse were receiving "the best medical care available in the United States" at that time.[25]

In addition, the periodic epidemics at Calverton provided fodder for early scientific studies, including an 1845 discourse on malaria patients there by William T. Howard, and Buckler's 1851 book, *History of Epidemic Cholera as It Appeared at the Baltimore City and County Almshouse in the Summer of 1849.*[26]

In 1853, Baltimore City and Baltimore County became separate political entities, and nine years later the city enacted an ordinance providing for the purchase from the Canton Company of a new Almshouse location. Once again, the Almshouse was to be situated far outside existing city limits, on a crest east of the city line overlooking the Chesapeake Bay. Baltimore bought 46 acres initially, later increasing its holdings to 240 acres, and spent more than $500,000 on a new three-story facility with symmetric wings that spanned 714 feet (twice the length of Calverton). The building was distinguished by an impressive domed rotunda; the dome's light served as a landmark for sailors on the Chesapeake Bay and the Patapsco River.[27]

In 1866, the residents of the Calverton Almshouse were moved to the new "Baltimore Bay View Asylum." The "asylum" part of the name change reflected the institution's role as an insane asylum as well as a place for miscreants, the poor and those needing medical care. Over the next century, this structure underwent many alterations, including the removal of its dome in 1954 and the gutting of its interior to increase its capacity from three to five stories. It is still part of the Bayview campus and is known today as the Mason F. Lord Building. The weathervane that crowned the dome in 1866 was saved and still registers wind changes atop the tower that replaced the dome.[28]

The move to Bay View improved the care of those sent there, as did the advances in medical treatment compelled by the horrific conditions on battlefields and in hospitals that tended wounded soldiers of the Civil War, which had ended just the year before Bay View opened. New attention to sanitation and the control of infection became standard; rules were established for improving patient care; medical students were closely supervised by the resident physician and required to present medical histories and physical findings from their examinations, as well as keep detailed medical records. In 1871, the first paying patients were admitted.[29]

Bay View's management became the duty of the new, five-member Board of Trustees of the Poor, appointed by the city government.[30] Records are scant regarding the type of treatment provided to patients in this era. Diagnoses registered in the vague medical language of the time include "debauch" (attributed to 38 patients in 1871) or simply "fever," which might be classified "cerebral," "congestive" or "typhoid." In 1871, the Asylum spent $1.74 a week per patient on care, which that year's annual report compared "favorably" with the $6.51 per week spent by the Pennsylvania Hospital or the $12.70 per week lavished on the patients at Massachusetts General Hospital. Hundreds of gallons of whiskey were purchased each year as a medication.[31]

In 1879, the Bay View trustees expressed growing alarm over the continuous and worsening overcrowding in the institution's inadequate facility for the insane and urged the state to do more to provide for these individuals.[32] This was to remain a problem for decades.

The plight of the insane residents of Bay View was among the factors that brought the facility to the attention of William H. Welch (1850-1934), the first professor of pathology at the new Johns Hopkins School of Medicine, when he arrived in Baltimore in 1885. Thus began the 120-year association between Hopkins and its future Eastern Avenue sibling. Welch, appointed to the Hopkins faculty in 1884, needed subjects for his students to study (The Johns Hopkins Hospital building itself would not open until 1889), and Welch's assistant, William Thomas Councilman (1854-1933), had been a pathologist at Bay View Asylum since 1879.[33] Councilman and other Hopkins physicians became visitors at Bay View. By 1886, the staffing of Bay View's hospital for the insane was undertaken by Hopkins, its records were organized, younger physicians were enlisted to join its staff, and medical students were taught there.[34]

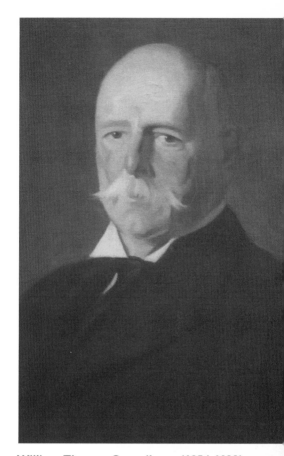

William Thomas Councilman (1854-1933), assistant to William Welch and pathologist at Bay View Asylum (1879), visiting physician to the insane wards at Bay View (1883-1892), Shattuck Professor of Pathology at the Harvard Medical School (1892). When he was Welch's assistant, he used a large tricycle to transport pathology specimens from Bay View to Hopkins—and sometimes accidentally dropped them in the street while en route. (MedChi, The Maryland State Medical Society)

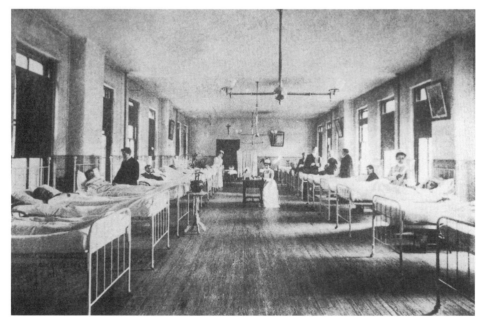

A ward in the Bay View Asylum, circa 1900. (HBBMS)

Sir William Osler, in bowler hat, visits Bay View Asylum in 1913. Left to right in this unfortunately damaged photo: **Thomas Boggs**, chief of medicine at Bay View and the former student at Johns Hopkins to whom Osler had given his stethoscope; **Osler**; **Thomas B. Futcher**, another protégé of Osler's who became a member of the Hopkins School of Medicine faculty; **Arthur Shipley**, Bay View's surgeon in chief, (alas, only partially visible). Boggs and Shipley ran Bay View for 27 years. (HBBMS)

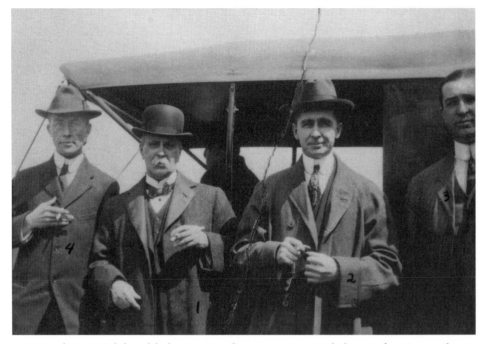

Years later, Welch told those attending a testimonial dinner for Councilman that in his early years as a pathologist, his younger colleague "had no pathological material save that which he obtained outside [of the new Hopkins medical school]. He purchased a tricycle and had occasional accidents which even got into the newspapers when the street was littered with specimens that escaped from the container attached to the tricycle."[35]

Councilman, who became a professor of pathology at the Harvard Medical School, was acclaimed for his studies of the pathological lesions produced by malarial fever. His observations at Bay View were the first in the United States to confirm the discovery by Nobel Prize-winning French pathologist Charles Louise Alphonse Laveran of the malarial parasite.[36] He also was known for his findings on the effects of yellow fever on the livers of patients dying of the disease. (One of Councilman's immediate successors as head of the Pathology Laboratory at Bay View was George H. Whipple [1878-1976], also a protégé of Welch, who obtained his medical degree from Hopkins in 1905. Whipple, who became dean of the School of Medicine and Dentistry at the University of Rochester, later won a Nobel Prize himself for his research on the etiology and therapy of pernicious anemia.[37])

The 1890s witnessed a revolution in medical education largely instituted by Johns Hopkins, which was aided in its mission by the proximity of Bay View. Although the Hopkins School of Medicine initially used Bay View as a source of pathological specimens and for the teaching of psychiatry, soon Hopkins' development of a system of student and residency training was adopted at Bay View as well, and Hopkins medical students began examining a wide range of Bay View patients.[38] Hopkins, the University of Maryland Medical School, and the College of Physicians and Surgeons (now

Mercy Hospital) nominated residents, assistant residents and medical students to the Bay View trustees for assignment there, and sent one or more of their own physicians to Bay View every day to tend to its patients.[39]

In 1890, Bay View established separate wards for treating patients with pulmonary tuberculosis. This innovation probably created the first separate tuberculosis wards ever in a general hospital in the United States, according to Edmund G. Beacham, long the chief of the tuberculosis division.[40] By 1893, the trustees' annual report separated information on medical and surgical cases for the first time, indicating improvements in the accuracy and details of diagnoses.[41] In 1896, the trustee report noted that management of the Asylum was being handled on a more businesslike basis; and in 1897, a city ordinance for the first time restricted the power of police magistrates to send vagrants and alcoholics to the Asylum, thus permitting the institution to focus its mission even more on medical treatment.[42]

With the opening of the tuberculosis ward, the need for trained nurses became more pressing. Since its founding as an almshouse, Bay View had relied on matrons to manage its daily activities and perform rudimentary nursing services, but in 1896, its annual report declared that "a competent trained nurse with an experienced assistant matron" had been hired, and noted that the "efficiency of the nursing corps had greatly increased through the installation at its head of a graduate nurse."[43]

In 1900, the new Baltimore City Charter replaced the Trustees of the Poor with the nine-member Board of Supervisors of City Charities, appointed by the mayor. The supervisors continued efforts to limit the police courts' power to send "beats and bums" to Bay View, which the supervisors argued could no longer be considered either a penal institution or a reformatory.[44] Despite Bay View's increasing concentration on medical care, it remained what one chronicler called the "catch-all for the petty thief, the vagrant, the penniless widow, the worn-out laborer, the insane, and the chronic invalid, who were sent there by various agencies of the city, and the patients the other hospitals didn't want."[45] (City magistrates retained the power to commit vagrants to Bay View until 1935, when the Maryland General Assembly ended the practice. The housing of indigent mental patients became the main responsibility of state mental hospitals in 1943.[46])

In December 1904, treatment for tuberculosis patients expanded with the opening of the Municipal Tuberculosis Hospital on the Bay View site, with

The Osler-Boggs stethoscope, now preserved in Osler's former study in The Johns Hopkins Hospital's Billings Administration Building. (The Alan Mason Chesney Medical Archives of The Johns Hopkins Medical Institutions)

accommodations for 170 patients. Within five years, 588 patients were being treated there at a daily cost of 49 cents per patient. (The number of TB patients at Bay View reached its peak in 1914, when 700 were treated there and 239 died.[47])

Baltimore Mayor J. Barry Mahool appointed a committee of municipal and medical leaders in 1909 to study the situation at the Asylum and propose improvements. The committee's recommendations led to growth and improvement at the Bay View Asylum, which accelerated significantly in 1911 with the opening of a new, state-of-the-art hospital building for the medical and surgical wards, a Y-shaped structure that eventually became the south wing of the facility's B Building. The same year also saw the appointments of two men who would guide the institution for the next 27 years: Thomas R. Boggs, chief of medicine from 1911 to 1938, and Arthur M. Shipley, surgeon in chief from 1911 to 1939.[48]

Both Boggs and Shipley were highly regarded leaders in their fields, and they opened a new era for Bay View. Under them, it was transformed into a modern hospital.

Thomas Boggs had served a 10-year residency at The Johns Hopkins Hospital and was, in fact, the young physician with whom the legendary Sir William Osler had gone on his last rounds at Hopkins in 1905 before handing over his stethoscope with the instruction, "Now carry on my work." (That stethoscope since has been returned to Hopkins Hospital and now rests in a display case inside the room in the domed administration building where Osler wrote his classic textbook, *The Principles and Practice of Medicine.*)

Boggs would more than honor Osler's charge, becoming an associate professor of medicine at Hopkins the same year he was appointed head of medicine at Bay View. A superior bedside teacher whose style closely emulated Osler's in

Bay View Infectious Diseases Building, 1909. The hospital had no X-ray equipment until 1919, and X-rays of Bay View patients that were taken at Hopkins Hospital or the University of Maryland Hospital took a day to be delivered via the horse-drawn "ambulance" seen in front of the building. (Baltimore *News American* photo, Special Collections, University of Maryland Libraries. ©The Hearst Corporation.)

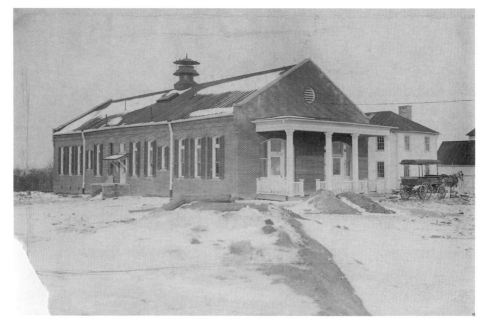

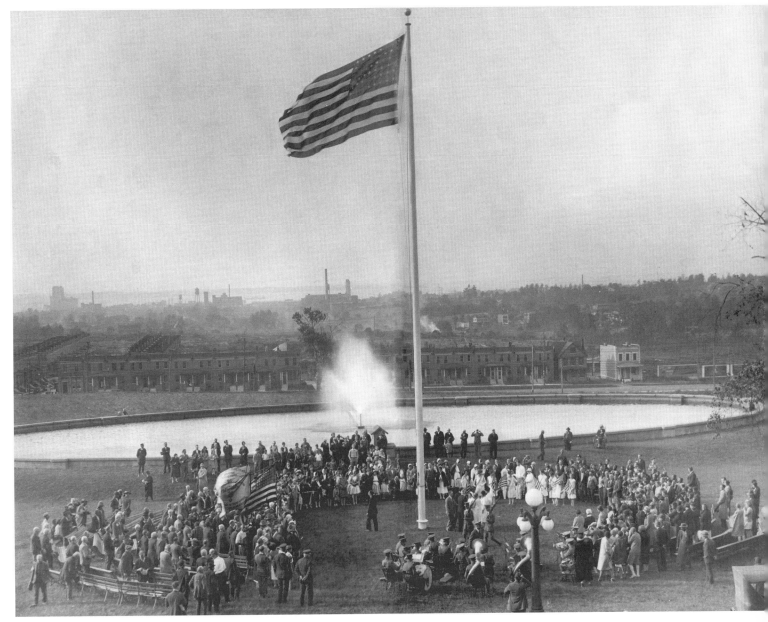

Flag-raising ceremony on City Hospitals' Eastern Avenue front lawn in 1929. (HBBMS)

its combination of scholarship, general knowledge and charm, Boggs conducted daily clinics that were attended eagerly by house officers. Widely known and respected by leaders in internal medicine elsewhere, Boggs' position greatly enhanced the institution's nationwide reputation. He became president of the Association of American Physicians in 1937.[49]

Arthur Shipley had been a member of Mayor Mahool's committee and superintendent of the University of Maryland Hospital, where he had reorganized the surgical service and helped modernize its medical school. He was president of the Baltimore Medical Society the year he was appointed surgeon in chief at Bay View and directed to reorganize its surgical service. A superb diagnostician and surgeon, he also maintained a private practice. The training program he offered attracted top-notch young physicians from around the country.[50]

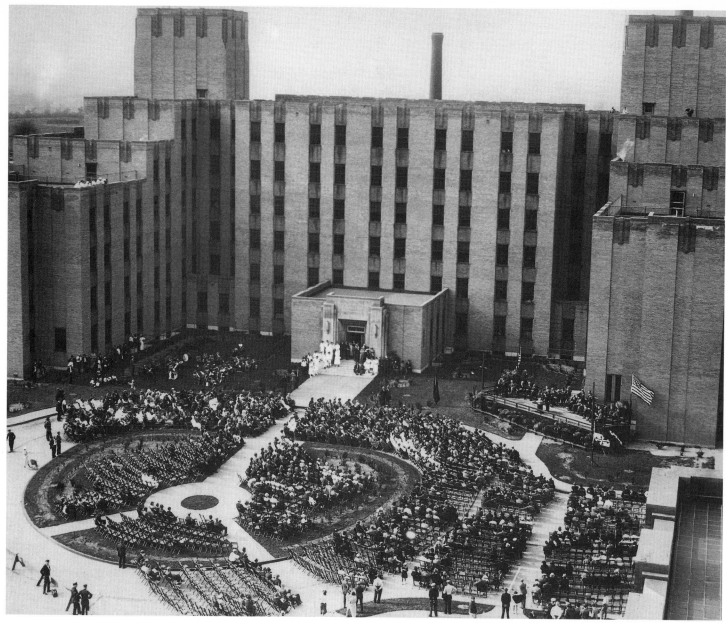

Grand opening in 1935 of City Hospitals' acute care building, now known as the **A Building, was presided over by Maryland's four-term Governor Albert C. Ritchie (1876-1936) (right), for whom Ritchie Highway is named. (HBBMS)**

The appointments of Boggs and Shipley created a custom under which the chiefs of medicine at Bay View came from the Hopkins faculty and the chiefs of surgery came from the University of Maryland faculty. This unwritten understanding was upheld for the next 45 years.[51]

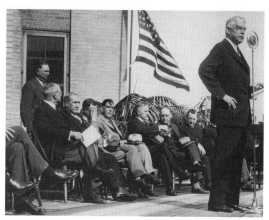

Under Boggs and Shipley, medical care was separated into five services: medicine, headed by Boggs; surgery, headed by Shipley; tuberculosis, headed by Gordon Wilson; pathology, headed by Milton C. Winternitz; and psychiatry, headed by Esther Richards. To alleviate a nursing shortage, a nurses' training school also opened in October 1911.

Despite these important appointments and the opening of the new tuberculosis facility and acute care hospital building within the first dozen years of the 20th century, the physicians at Bay View Asylum still had to deal with a frustratingly parsimonious city. In 1913, the three hospitals on the Asylum grounds—the infirmary, the tuberculosis sanitarium and the acute care hospital—still had only one telephone among them, and no switchboard. Requests for X-ray equipment made in 1912 were ignored for six years, despite the fact that it took an entire day for a horse-drawn ambulance to deliver the X-rays of Bay View patients taken at Hopkins or University hospitals. When X-ray equipment finally was ordered for Bay View in 1918, it could not be used for another year because the $75-a-month salary of a technician to operate it had been lopped from the budget.[52]

The entry of the United States into World War I in April 1917 led to the military enlistment of many physicians, including Boggs, Shipley and Wilson.[53] Winternitz left to become a professor of pathology at Yale Medical School, of which he eventually became dean.[54] Because of the acute shortage of doctors during the war, fourth-year medical students took the place of many attending physicians at the hospitals.

Doctors Boggs and Shipley returned to Bay View in 1919 after the war's end and embarked on a long battle to increase funding, enhance the medical care provided, and improve facilities that had been allowed to deteriorate drastically for want of city support. This was due largely to the woeful indifference of the increasingly politicized Board of Supervisors of City Charities, composed mostly of "minor politicians chiefly concerned with peanut jobs which had some relation to the purchase of supplies for the 1,500 or 1,800 helpless paupers and lunatics" at Bay View, wrote *The Sun's* Mark S. Watson.[55]

By 1923, the lower floor of the original 1866 building resembled a medieval prison. C. Holmes Boyd, then a third-year Hopkins medical student, recalled decades later that although the "halls of the main floor were black and white marble, beneath at ground level were brick vaulted cellars frequently dripping moisture, reminding one of dungeons of another era, and in which lived some of the inmates."[56] Bay View, Boyd wrote, was "feared as a Black Hole of Calcutta and people fought against being sent there." The often appalling conditions in which the mentally ill were housed led the public to associate the name "Bay View" with insanity—and hopelessness. Baltimore mothers were known to throw a scare into recalcitrant children by threatening that if they didn't behave, they'd be sent to Bay View.[57]

"No words in the English language can describe the conditions at the institution when I arrived," said Colonel (later Brigadier General) Rufus E. Longan, who was appointed superintendent of Bay View in 1923 after a raucous and explosive board of supervisors meeting at which seven of the nine members abruptly resigned.[58] A newly organized board undertook a wide search to find an experienced administrator and quickly settled on Longan, who had

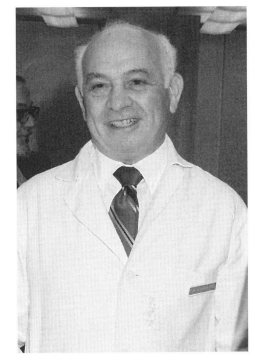

Harold Harrison (1908-1989) was the first full-time chief of the department of pediatrics at Baltimore City Hospitals, holding that post from 1945 to 1975. His collaboration with City Hospitals colleague Laurence Finberg on preventing diarrhea in babies, which led to the development of oral rehydration therapy, still saves an estimated one million infants a year worldwide. Harrison was instrumental in developing the hospital's medical library, which now houses his papers and bears his name. (HBBMS)

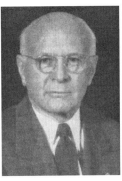

Parker J. McMillin (1888-1972) became the first professional hospital administrator to be appointed superintendent of City Hospitals in 1934. He led the hospital throughout the Depression, World War II and the 1950s, retiring in 1959. (HBBMS)

The latest medical equipment of 1935 was available in the X-ray department, the women's ward, and the pediatric ward housed in the new City Hospitals building. (HBBMS)

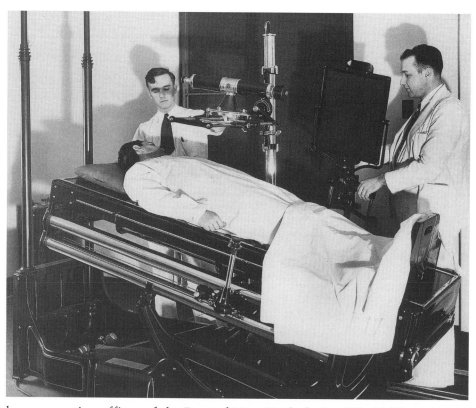

been executive officer of the Port of New York during World War I.

An out-of-towner unconcerned with local ward heeler politics, Longan was appalled by what he found at Bay View. "The buildings were in a woeful state of repair. The power plant was a wreck. The human element was also a wreck. The stench and smells that prevailed were indescribable. The food was extremely poor. It was all due to negligence. [I]t was a place for putting political henchmen to work. Housing conditions were rotten. There was a shortage of help and the help on hand was not of the proper quality. There was less than an average of one blanket per patient. Bedding was unfit to use. All of this had to be replaced."[59]

In addition to implementing money-saving improvements (such as scrapping an ancient heating system and installing a new one that saved $14,000 a year) and opening the Training School of Practical Nursing in 1925, Longan also sought to alter the institution's image by changing its name. In 1925, the Bay View Asylum was rechristened the Baltimore City Hospitals.[60] The plural "Hospitals" reflected the fact that multiple hospitals existed on the same site for acute care, chronic care and tuberculosis.[61] Dropping "Asylum" from the name was an effort to erase the stigma that had become associated with it. The name change also reflected that fewer insane patients were being treated there, since many of them were being sent to new state mental hospitals, and that more medical care was being provided to poor patients in the wards and the outpatient department.[62]

The name change did not alter the grim realities in the inadequately

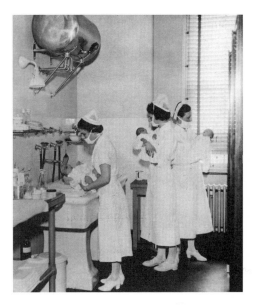

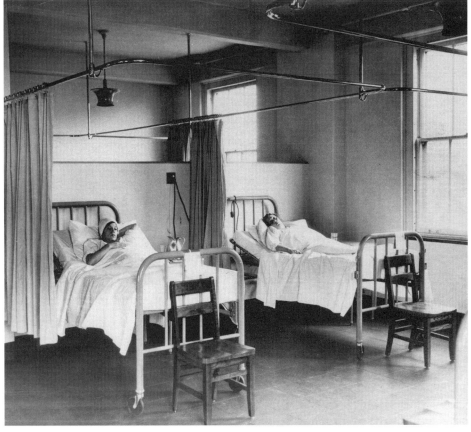

funded, perennially neglected facilities. In 1926, Boggs and Shipley issued a somber report: "The Chronic Wards have been expanded beyond the limits of propriety and strict honesty. This situation is an urgent reality. It is impossible to maintain morale. First and last the solution lies in adequate personnel, adequately paid." The following year, the hospitals' staff pointed out that Baltimore paid less per day for the care of its indigent patients than any large city in the nation.[63]

By 1929, at the urging of both The Johns Hopkins University and the University of Maryland and with the assistance of Winford Smith, director of Hopkins hospital, as architectural consultant (donating services for which he might have been paid $55,000), Baltimore City completed plans to erect a new general hospital, tuberculosis sanitarium, service building and nurses' home at City Hospitals.[64] Surprisingly, despite the stock market crash and subsequent Great Depression, Baltimore fulfilled those plans. New living quarters for some 110 nurses then training and working at City Hospitals opened in 1931. A new 450-bed general hospital, the present-day A Building, opened in 1935, as did the north section of the B Building. A new tuberculosis sanitarium opened in 1937.[65]

Overseeing much of this construction and modernization was Parker J. McMillin (1888-1972), who succeeded Longan in 1934 and became the first professional hospital administrator to be appointed superintendent of City

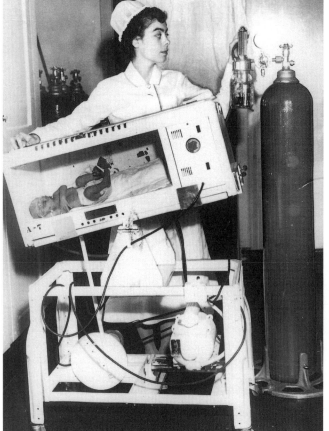

The "Rocker Incubator" was a City Hospitals' baby-boom innovation. Designed in 1953 by two renowned pediatricians, Harold Harrison and Laurence Finberg, with funds contributed by the Highlandtown Exchange Club, this device provided artificial respiration for premature infants via a constant seesaw motion. "A motor, belt, fly-wheel and rocker-arm tilt the incubator and junior 20 to 25 times a minute," explained *The Sun*. (Photograph by Frank P. Kalita, ©1953 *The Baltimore Sun*. Used by permission.)

Hospitals, following a nationwide search for an experienced manager. McMillin, who spent the next quarter century running City Hospitals, was a native of Lancaster, Ohio. He had only a high school diploma, plus some brief commercial coursework. Yet within three years of joining the purchasing department of the Ford Motor Company in Detroit in 1912, he rose to become purchasing agent for the Henry Ford Hospital. By 1918, at the age of 30, he was named its superintendent. Three years later, McMillin was named superintendent of the Cleveland City Hospital, one of the largest municipal hospitals in the country. He was there when Baltimore recruited him 13 years later to head City Hospitals.[66]

Working closely with Boggs and Shipley, who were only part-time administrators at City Hospitals, McMillin maintained the momentum to remake the facilities through the depths of the Depression. He also fought and eventually won the battle to have mental patients removed from City Hospitals and treated in state-run hospitals instead. (Although the state formally assumed responsibility for the care of the insane in 1911, for more than 30 years it made no effort to accommodate mental patients already housed at City Hospitals, the last of whom remained until 1943.[67])

That Boggs, Shipley and McMillin were a powerful team is evidenced by the impressive investment Baltimore made in medical care of the poor at City Hospitals, which had become part of city government in 1934 when a city charter amendment abolished the Board of Supervisors of City Charities and created the Department of Public Welfare. The hospital became part of the new welfare department. Judge Thomas J.S. Waxter, the new department's first director, was a forceful advocate for the hospitals and for proper medical care for poor Baltimoreans.[68]

Boggs died in 1938 and was succeeded by John T. King. In 1939, Shipley retired and was succeeded by Thomas B. Alcock. The impact that Boggs and Shipley had on City Hospitals had been profound. Along with their colleagues, they sought to ensure that superior bedside medicine was practiced at City Hospitals; and they made the professional training and personal success of their house staffs a top priority. Their reputation was such that "[y]oung doctors from across the United States came to work at the Baltimore City Hospitals," Carroll wrote.[69]

In addition to Judge Waxter, important allies of Boggs, Shipley and Parker McMillin included George Walker, a prominent Baltimore urologist who was on City Hospitals' board of trustees, and Alan Chesney, dean of The Johns Hopkins School of Medicine. Both of these men worked to enhance the relationship between City Hospitals and the Hopkins and University of Maryland medical schools. City Hospitals' staff physicians were appointed to the faculties of both medical schools, and patients at City

Hospitals were used in teaching the universities' medical students.[70]

City Hospitals' building boom of the 1930s was the capstone to the careers of Boggs and Shipley—and the last major investment in its physical plant for some 20 years. Closer ties with the city's major medical schools endured, however, and other enhancements and innovations continued, including the creation of full-time positions for physicians to head various hospital services. In 1937, Frank Kendall, for years a resident in pathology at The Johns Hopkins Hospital, was appointed pathologist in chief at City Hospitals, making him the first full-time chief of a service there. And in 1940, King succeeded in persuading the U.S. Public Health Service to establish a small research unit of one technician and one researcher within the hospital's new Department of Gerontology, headed by Edward J. Stieglitz. In 1941, Nathan Shock joined this department and began developing programs that in time became world-famous. From this seedling would grow a substantial institutional specialty in the study of and caring for the aging.[71]

In December 1941, the entry of the United States into World War II halted improvements at City Hospitals. Skyrocketing wartime wages in private industry outstripped the municipal salaries available at the hospitals, and many support employees left. The nursing staff, plagued by recurring cycles of abundance during lean financial times and shortage during prosperous ones, dipped drastically as nurses began enrolling in the Army Nurses' Corps Reserve and many nursing schools shut down. City Hospitals, which had closed its nurses' training school as a cost-cutting measure in 1934, opened the new School of Practical Nursing in 1941. By 1943, City Hospitals was the only general hospital in Maryland with a program in practical nursing.[72]

Simply keeping City Hospitals up and running during the war was a major challenge.[73] The number of visiting physicians and house staff declined as doctors entered the military; the nursing shortage remained desperate. In 1942, some 1,550 patients were turned away because of the staffing shortage, and only 161 registered nurses and nurses' aides did the work that 295 nurses and aides had handled in 1939.[74] Ironically, immediately after the war, the personnel crisis at City Hospitals got worse still when the conscientious objectors and German prisoners who had been assigned to work there as support staff left in 1946.[75]

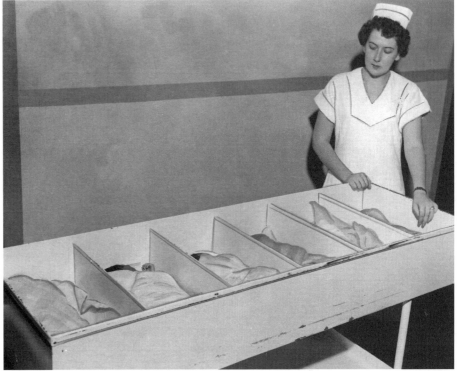

Another baby-boom innovation of the postwar years at City Hospitals was this baby cart, cobbled together for transporting many infants to their mothers for feeding. Recalls Philip Zieve: "We, as medical students, delivered a lot of babies without much supervision, and the babies came at a terrific rate." (Baltimore *News American* photo, Special Collections, University of Maryland Libraries. ©The Hearst Corporation.)

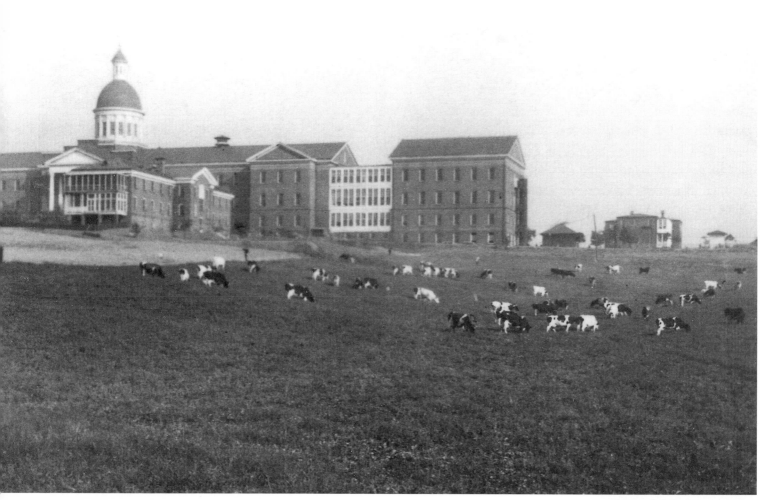

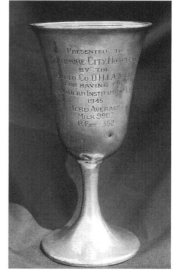

City Hospitals' dairy cows graze beside the main, 1866 building. Right, a cup awarded to the hospital for its superior milk production in 1945. Farming operations at City Hospitals ceased in 1948, ending the last of the workhouse functions of the original Almshouse. The inscription on the cup cites the herd's average production that year as 9,907 pounds of milk per cow, with a butterfat content of 36.2 percent. (HBBMS)

These wartime personnel problems demonstrated convincingly that the most effective way to operate City Hospitals was to have full-time chiefs head each department, not part-time doctors with outside commitments. In 1945, Harold Harrison became the first full-time chief in the department of pediatrics; Frederick Mandeville was named full-time chief of the X-ray department; and Gardner Warner was selected to be the full-time chief of pathology.[76]

The wartime funding drought ended in 1948, when Baltimore city voters passed an $8 million bond issue for improvements at City Hospitals, including renovation of the acute care hospital and construction of a new tuberculosis unit. The focus on pure medicine was symbolized by the discontinuation in 1948 of the hospital's farming operations, including its award-winning dairy herd, a fixture at the site since Bay View opened in 1866. It was the last remnant of the institution's days as an almshouse where poor people worked for their keep.[77]

In 1952, the positions of physician in chief and three assistant chiefs were made full-time, setting the stage for a more active teaching program at both undergraduate and graduate levels. Among those selected for these positions was C. Holmes Boyd (who had remembered the dripping catacombs in the infirmary during the 1920s) as chief of medicine. The participation of medical students grew dramatically, research activities were initiated, and City Hospitals' quality of care improved.[78] Later, in 1954, Edmund G. Beacham became chief of the tuberculosis division. Beacham was a native Baltimorean, accomplished lacrosse player and decorated veteran of World War II who began his association with City Hospitals as an intern in 1940 following his graduation from the University of Maryland School of Medicine. He would remain a leader at the institution for more than 40 years.[79]

In the late 1940s and early 1950s, Harold Harrison's research on preventing diarrhea in babies led him to devise a method of oral rehydration therapy about which he published a paper in 1954. Later, the famed British medical journal, *The Lancet*, proclaimed the therapy "potentially the most important medical advance this century." It is estimated that one million infants a year still are saved by treatment derived from Harrison's research.[80]

By 1955, third-year medical students from Johns Hopkins were receiving about half of their practical experience in medicine at City Hospitals, serving as clinical clerks there.[81] Among the University of Maryland medical students who arrived at City Hospitals for rotations in obstetrics and chronic medicine in 1956 was Philip Zieve, who would join the staff in 1964, become an internationally recognized hematologist and serve as chairman of the department of medicine and elected chief of the professional staff for more than 20 years.

The "chronic hospital" that Zieve saw for the first time in 1956 was, he says, "a museum of medical and neurological curiosities," a repository of several hundred patients who had lived there at city expense for as long as half a century—since Theodore Roosevelt's presidency. The facility and its inmates essentially served as instructional tools for Hopkins and Maryland medical students. "It was mainly warehousing," Zieve recalls. "Very little was done to help these people, although if they developed acute, inter-current illness, they were treated. And our function there was mainly not to help at all with the service requirements but to do histories and physical exams under supervision. The hospital was proud of the fact that [the patients] rarely got pressure sores, because of a dedicated nursing service."[82]

In obstetrics, Zieve became immersed in what was said at the time to be the busiest baby-birthing service in the nation. "I can't remember how many deliveries there were here, but we, as medical students, delivered a lot

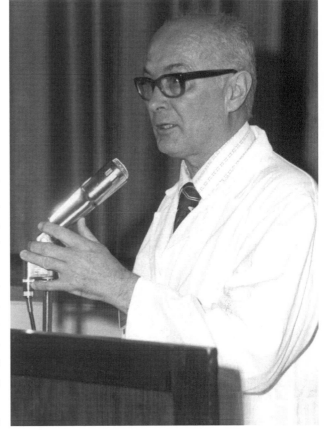

Edmund G. Beacham, seen here in a 1970s photo, began his distinguished medical career at Baltimore City Hospitals in 1941, serving in succession as chief of the tuberculosis department and chief of chronic and community medicine and of chronic medicine and geriatrics. When he began his career, "most of the care we gave was relatively free of cost," he recalls. "This was a municipal hospital, and those who came generally couldn't afford to pay or paid very little." In the 1970s, he began an annual geriatrics symposium that attracted hundreds of physicians from around the nation. The Beacham Ambulatory Care Center and Beacham Adult Day Care Center at Hopkins Bayview are named in his honor. He retired in 1984 and became emeritus consultant in geriatric medicine at The Johns Hopkins University School of Medicine. (HBBMS)

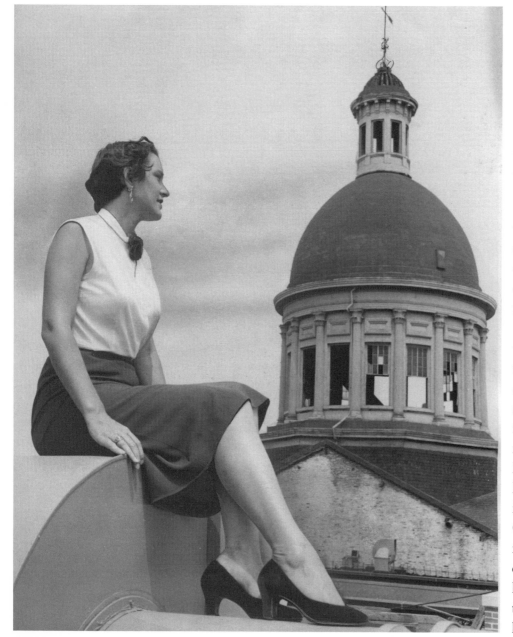

A classic 1950s newspaper photo features a City Hospitals employee taking the air as the old Bay View Asylum dome is readied for dismantling. Assigned to take a picture of the doomed dome, Baltimore *News American* photographer Vernon Price decided that a person would enliven the shot. (Baltimore *News American* photo, Special Collections, University of Maryland Libraries. ©The Hearst Corporation.)

of babies without much supervision, and the babies came at a terrific rate." The baby boom was in full swing, and there was no Medicaid program yet, so poor mothers had few places to go for no-cost delivery service, Zieve notes. City Hospitals took care of many poor mothers from outside Baltimore.[83]

Baltimore was allocating $3,585,000 to operate City Hospitals, of which only $350,000 was recovered by billing patients who lived outside the city or were admitted as emergency cases, then found to be insured or otherwise able to pay. "The operating costs compare favorably with those of other hospitals," McMillin wrote in a 1955 article for the *Maryland State Medical Journal,* noting that by "caring for the indigent residents of Baltimore, [the] original purpose of the hospital is being respected and adhered to."[84] Yet with the growth of its teaching and research programs, City Hospitals also had been transformed into "a modern medical center," McMillin, affectionately known as "Mr. Mac," confidently told *The Sun* when he announced his intention to retire in 1959.[85]

In fact, City Hospitals struck Chester W. Schmidt Jr., a Johns Hopkins medical student who arrived there in 1959, as far from modern. In reality, it was a "very decrepit, run-down, primitive" place, "bursting at the seams with patients." All the wards were open; hanging cloth dividers separated the beds, which were lined up in long corridors, spaced perhaps 10 feet apart. "All of the blood tests, urinalysis, mixing of bodily fluids, bacteriology, was done by hand by the medical students and the house staff, without any sense of the quality control of laboratories today," Schmidt recalls with a bemused smile.[86] Schmidt, a native New Yorker, later completed his residency in psychiatry at the Henry Phipps Psychiatric Clinic at Hopkins. Appointed chief of the department of psychiatry at City Hospitals in 1972, he would be elected

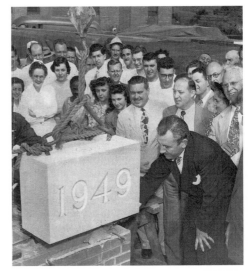

Baltimore Mayor Thomas D'Alesandro Jr. presides over installation of the cornerstone at City Hospitals' new tuberculosis unit in 1949. This building and an ensuing renovation of the acute care hospital were the first construction projects on the campus since the 1930s. (HBBMS)

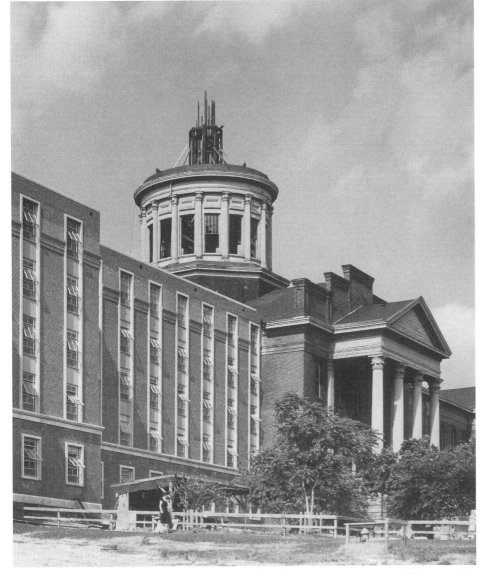

The dome on the original 1866 Bay View Asylum Almshouse building was demolished in August 1954. It had topped what was then called the D Building and is now the Mason F. Lord Building. The weathervane on the old dome was saved, put atop its replacement tower, and still signals wind changes on Eastern Avenue after nearly 140 years. (©1954 *The Baltimore Sun.* Used by permission.)

president of the hospitals' pioneering faculty practice group, Chesapeake Physicians Professional Association (CPPA), in 1977 and remain its head for more than 25 years.[87]

Despite the conditions Zieve and Schmidt observed in the late 1950s, by 1960 the local press was heralding the "transformation" of City Hospitals since the end of World War II. In contrast to the dearth of full-time physicians in 1945, the hospital had 33 full-time doctors by 1960, including "men of international reputation," *The Sun* proclaimed. Harrison was the recipient of a gold medal from the American Academy of Pediatrics and its $1,000 Borden Prize. Nathan Shock, the chief of research gerontology who had begun his work at City Hospitals in 1941, was chosen by *Modern Medicine* magazine as one of the 10 outstanding biological scientists of 1960. Mark N. Ravitch, chief of the department of surgery, was an editor of both *Surgery* magazine and *The Quarterly Review of Surgery.* Francis Chinard, head of the Department of

Grim conditions inside the City Hospitals' infirmary are illustrated in this 1951 photo taken for the old *Evening Sun.* A forlorn resident of a six-bed room sits near dangerously crumbling plaster, which required the removal of two beds from beside the decaying wall. "The room is very dingy and badly lighted," the photographer noted on the back of the picture. (Photograph by William Klender, ©1951 *The Baltimore Sun.* Used by permission.)

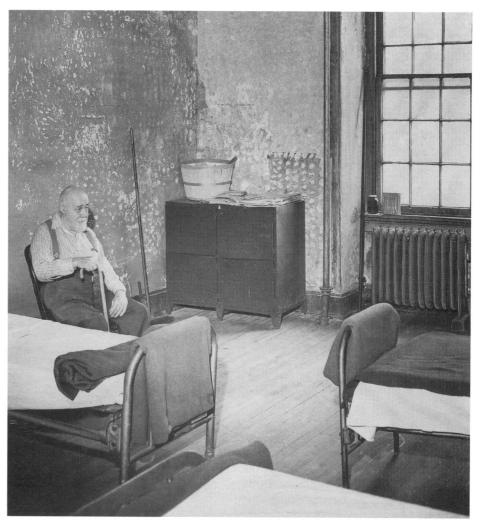

Medicine, was elected to the prestigious New York Academy of Sciences and served as an editor of *The American Journal of Physiology* and the *Journal of Applied Physiology.*[88]

Notwithstanding the impressive accomplishments of City Hospitals' physicians, the physical plant of the late 1950s was becoming outdated. As late as 1961, its large, open wards provided little patient privacy and lacked proper plumbing facilities, call systems and air conditioning. Major modernization efforts were called for, but only a few modest ones were undertaken, and archaic peculiarities were left intact.[89]

"When McMillin was here, the acute hospital, which was built in the early '30s [and] had the acute medical, surgical and pediatric services, had a third floor that was called 'A-4.' The fourth floor was called 'A-3.' The fifth floor was called 'A-7'," recalls Zieve with a chuckle. The decidedly quirky floor designations followed no apparent logic, but according to Zieve, McMillin "could not bring himself to change those to their appropriate levels because he said it had always been done that way and people wouldn't understand it if it were changed. That's how he ran the hospital."[90]

Toward the end of his tenure, McMillin persuaded the city to seek a $3.5 million loan for some modernization and expansion of City Hospitals.[91] Under his successor, superintendent (later executive director) Frederick G. Hubbard, these funds were used to begin erecting an addition to the acute care hospital to house the department of anesthesiology, clinical laboratories, new operating rooms, the obstetrical delivery suite, premature and well-baby units and other facilities. This addition was completed in 1965, as were a group of garden apartments for the hospitals' house staff. A new $8 million research building for the gerontological unit was begun in 1966.[92]

City Hospitals handled its last widespread outbreak of poliomyelitis in 1960, when it became the first hospital in the United States to eliminate use of the iron lung respirator in favor of using positive ventilation of the Moerch or Bennett type to create positive pressure ventilation. Peter Safar (1924-2003), the first full-time chief of anesthesiology at City Hospitals, oversaw the development of this treatment. Safar also pioneered mouth-to-mouth resuscitation, often modified by the use of a "Safar Airway," and cardiopulmonary resuscitation (CPR) in the early 1960s. His innovations earned him recognition as "the father of CPR." He modestly declined that honorific, but many thought he deserved it. His work defined CPR's essential ABCs: maintaining a patient's airway, breathing and circulation. He later collaborated with a Norwegian company to create the first CPR training mannequin, "Resusci Anne," well known now to all who have trained in lifesaving courses.[93]

In addition, Safar's development of positive pressure ventilation procedures for treating apneic patients led in 1958 to creation of City Hospitals' medical-surgical multidisciplinary intensive care unit, the first ICU in the country with 24-hour coverage by anesthesiologists. Patients from any service who had any acute disease could be admitted to it at the discretion of the house staff.[94]

Also in 1958, under the leadership of Nathan Shock and Reuben Andres, the Gerontology Research Center's Clinical Physiology Branch began the Baltimore Longitudinal Study, a unique project that has gathered clinical, biochemical, physiological and psychological data on the aging process in hundreds of Baltimore residents over the past four decades.[95] Another innovation of this period was the introduction of a

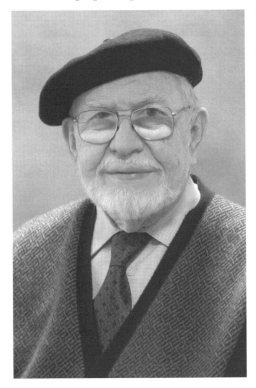

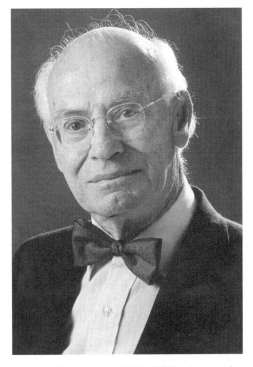

Nathan W. Shock (1906-1989) above, the dean of American gerontology, was director of the Gerontology Research Center on the Bayview campus for 35 years. Along with **Reuben Andres**, left, he founded the Baltimore Longitudinal Study of Aging (BLSA) in 1958 and was instrumental in developing and organizing various governmental and scientific societies devoted to advancing the study of human aging. After nearly 50 years, the BLSA continues to gather clinical, biochemical, physiological and psychological data on hundreds of Baltimore residents who have participated in the study for decades. (HBBMS)

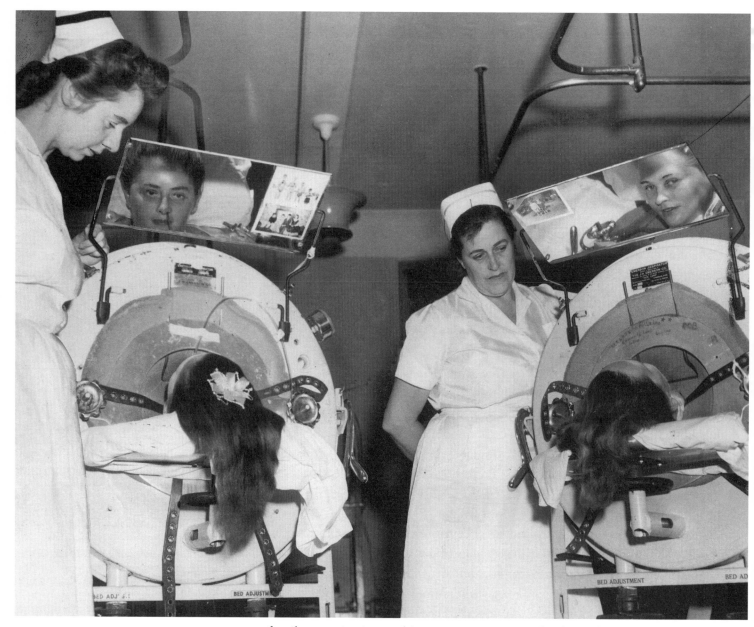

Iron lung respirators still were in use at City Hospitals in 1959, when this photo appeared in the old *News-Post and Sunday American.* The hospital handled its last widespread outbreak of poliomyelitis in 1960, and became the first hospital in the United States to eliminate use of iron lungs in favor of positive pressure ventilation treatment, overseen by Peter Safar. (Baltimore *News American* photo, Special Collections, University of Maryland Libraries. ©The Hearst Corporation.)

family practice internship program—again, the first of its kind in the country—under the direction of George S. Mirick, Francis Chinard, Harold E. Harrison and John O. Neustadt. It enabled physicians to deal with patients from infancy to old age, with an emphasis on pediatrics, internal medicine and psychiatry.[96] And in 1962, City Hospitals' cancer chemotherapy unit, which Albert Owens had begun with a few beds in the tuberculosis hospital, was moved to the B Building. It would provide the foundation for oncology research and treatment at The Johns Hopkins Hospital.

"The Johns Hopkins Hospital talks about its firsts. We've had a lot of firsts [at City Hospitals] that we haven't talked about a lot that I think stand up against those firsts," Zieve observes dryly. "Despite our impoverishment over the years, and our less-than-pretty face, we've done a lot, not only for the people that we serve but the people around the country, perhaps the world, who have benefited from the innovations that have been instituted here."[97]

In 1963, a new department of chronic and community medicine was created under the direction of Mason F. Lord (1926-1965), establishing a program for the long-term care of welfare patients with chronic diseases. Lord, the scion of a prominent Baltimore family, was a charismatic Renaissance man. An opera lover, he traveled often to the Spoleto Festival in Italy; formally "conducted" operas in his home, using records or radio broadcasts for the music; and would sing arias from "Rigoletto" to Italian patients or "Boris Godunov" to Russian patients. Lord also was an accomplished art collector and an elegantly attired, witty conversationalist who always wore a carnation in his lapel.[98]

"He was a tall, imperious, aristocratic-looking man, but he had a feeling for the elderly and the chronically ill, and he determined to devote his life to them. And he did," recalls Zieve, who considered Lord his mentor. Financially independent, Lord accepted the small salary that Baltimore paid to full-time members of City Hospitals' staff, but "he really didn't need the money and didn't do it for the money. He did it out of a humanitarian interest in the patient population," Zieve says.[99]

Lord's innovative concepts for geriatric care, involving application of the principles of preventive medicine to the treatment of the elderly, became prototypes for similar systems nationwide. By instituting an intensive program of early rehabilitation as a way to prevent elderly patients from becoming invalids, he managed to reduce the length of stay for patients in the chronic hospital; this shortened the average waiting period for admission to it from six months to several weeks. Lord also strove to create community-wide home care programs and to improve nursing homes.[100] His tragic death from a brain tumor at the age of 39 was widely mourned and led to the renaming of City Hospitals' original 1866 building in his honor.

In 1965, Baltimore's voters approved a charter change, separating City Hospitals from its three-decade association with the city's welfare department and creating a new city agency, the Department of Hospitals, to monitor City Hospitals' increasingly complex operations. This change in oversight reflected the hospitals' growth, which, combined with skyrocketing costs for medical care and an overwhelmed accounting staff, made management of the hospitals

The first intensive care unit in the United States to have 24-hour coverage by anesthesiologists opened in City Hospitals a year before this 1959 photo was taken. (Baltimore *News American* photo, Special Collections, University of Maryland Libraries. ©The Hearst Corporation.)

Peter Safar (1924-2003), the first full-time chief of anesthesiology at City Hospitals, demonstrates the "Safar Airway" and his new method for mouth-to-mouth resuscitation in 1957. His pioneering work in cardiopulmonary resuscitation, using medical student volunteers, earned him the title "Father of CPR." He also created the first modern intensive care unit in the United States at City Hospitals in 1958, formulated basic principles of emergency medicine, and contributed to the design of modern ambulances. He later became chairman of the University of Pittsburgh Medical Center's anesthesiology department and established what now is known as the Safar Center for Resuscitation Research. (Baltimore *News American* photo, Special Collections, University of Maryland Libraries. ©The Hearst Corporation.)

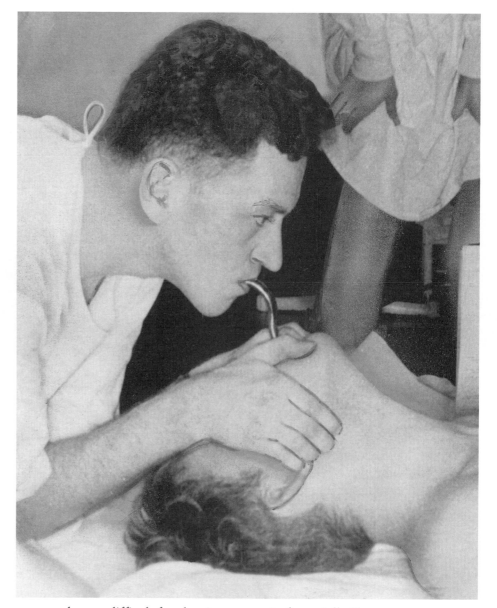

more and more difficult for the city to sustain financially.[101]

Despite its impending fiscal perils, City Hospitals managed to obtain city, state and federal funds to continue its growth and innovations. Some long-delayed renovations and expansions were undertaken in the mid-1960s. In June 1968, the federal government's National Institute on Aging completed building its new $7.5 million, four-story Gerontology Research Center at City Hospitals. When it opened with a staff of 130 investigators and support personnel, it was the world's largest research center on aging.[102] In November 1968, the Kiwanis Burn Unit, later the Baltimore Regional Burn Center, opened with the aid of a $20,000 contribution raised by the Kiwanis Club of Highlandtown (now the Kiwanis Club of East Baltimore) through rummage sales, newspaper ads, members' donations and a charity game by the Baltimore Bullets pro basketball team. Thomas Krizek, chief of plastic surgery at the hospital and a member of the Kiwanis, had challenged fellow club member Donald Hannahs during a bowling match in 1966 to see if the organization could raise the funds for the burn unit, which became the only one of its kind in Maryland.[103] Kiwanis not only met that challenge, but over the next 25 years donated more than $1 million to the center, which has treated thousands of burn patients from Maryland, Pennsylvania, Delaware and West Virginia.[104]

The first kidney transplant in Maryland—one of the first in the nation—was performed at City Hospitals in November 1968 by Richard Steenberg and Arnold Walder. Exactly a year later, in November 1969, the world's first heart pacemaker capable of being recharged under the skin was successfully implanted in a dog at City Hospitals by Kenneth B. Lewis, chief of cardiology at City Hospitals and an assistant professor of medicine at Hopkins. Powered by a nickel-cadmium battery, the new pacemaker, conceived by Robert E. Fischell at Johns Hopkins and developed by the Applied Physics Laboratory of The Johns Hopkins University, was a vast improvement over conventional pacemakers of the time, which had to be surgically removed in order to be recharged.[105]

Advances in the care of tuberculosis led to a rapid reduction in the need for hospital facilities to treat patients afflicted with the disease. By the late 1960s, only two major hospitals in Maryland treated TB patients: Mt. Wilson in Baltimore County and City Hospitals. In 1969, the state decided to consolidate treatment of TB patients at Mt. Wilson and closed Baltimore City Hospitals' pioneering tuberculosis division. Edmund Beacham, long-time chief of the TB division, became chief of the Division of Chronic and Community Medicine in 1970, renamed it the Division of Chronic Medical Care and oversaw a 301-bed facility for the treatment of patients requiring long-term rehabilitation due to strokes, arthritis, neurological and orthopedic problems and nutrition deficiencies.[106]

In July 1970, just a month after the chronic care division was launched, Medicare regulations compelled the reclassification of patients and the conditions for which they would receive federal medical coverage. Many patients thus became ineligible for subsidized care. Because Maryland's Medicaid payments were considerably lower than the actual costs of treatment, Baltimore

The first construction at City Hospitals in more than 15 years was celebrated in 1965, with the opening of an addition to the acute care hospital building. Harold Harrison addresses the audience at the building's dedication. Seated on the left in the light suit is City Council president Thomas J. D'Alesandro, III; to his left in a light suit is Mayor Theodore R. McKeldin; on the right, wearing glasses, is Frederick G. Hubbard, executive director of City Hospitals from 1959 to 1976. (HBBMS)

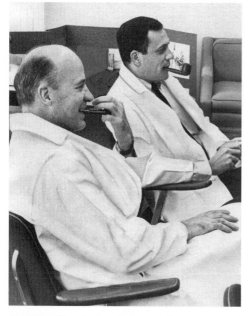

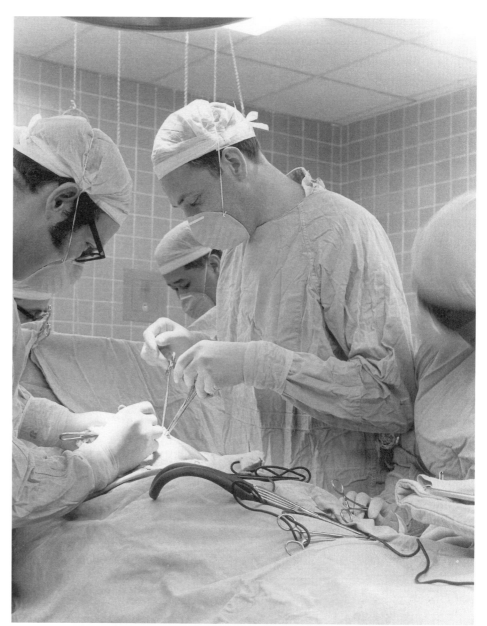

A City Hospitals photographer captured **Arnold Walder,** right, participating in the first kidney transplant in Maryland in November 1968. Above, Walder, right, and his co-surgeon in the pioneering procedure, **Richard Steenberg,** later discussed the successful operation with the press. (Above, Baltimore *News American* photo, Special Collections, University of Maryland Libraries. ©Hearst Corporation; right, HBBMS)

city anticipated sustaining a numbing $2.5 million deficit due to chronic medical care in 1971-72. Draconian economies were imposed. In July 1971, it was announced that the salaries the city paid to chronic care division physicians would be eliminated the following year, and the staff of nurses, social workers, rehabilitation aides and administrators was cut dramatically. Even the food service in the building was closed. The city agreed to keep the Chronic Medical Care Division open at a reduced patient level only if the deficit it incurred could be trimmed to $500,000 annually, a benchmark the division almost met by adhering to stringent budget restrictions.[107]

The costs of medical care grew exponentially as technology improved, particularly radiological and laboratory equipment, and as non-physician hospital staff began to organize and obtain much-needed salary increases.

Although Medicare and Medicaid payments were low, the programs at least assured steady payment for medical services—provided City Hospitals could manage to collect it, a task that proved beyond the capabilities of hospital administrators hired by the city.[108] City Hospitals' financial woes were inextricably linked not only to a city bureaucracy that could not manage a complex, modern medical facility, but also to the fiscal plight of Baltimore, which found itself mired in intractable social and budgetary crises by the early 1970s.

"The city of Baltimore ultimately was responsible for sending out bills and collecting the money. They didn't know how to do it and they did it poorly, so there was a lot of money left on the table," recalls Zieve. "They didn't know how to control expenses. They didn't know anything about hospital finances. So they had costs they didn't need to have, and they had revenue that they should have collected and didn't."[109]

Yet, even as Baltimore's politicians demanded cost-cutting at City Hospitals, they looked upon the facility as a cash cow from which the city could milk revenues by overcharging for such services as administration, financial management and insurance.[110]

Mason F. Lord (1926-1965) was the first full-time chief of chronic and community medicine at Baltimore City Hospitals (1963-1965). Lord devoted his career to developing programs for the comprehensive care of the chronically ill and aging by applying the principles of preventive medicine and rehabilitation, in the process establishing key principles of modern geriatrics. An art patron and music lover, he always wore a carnation on his lapel. (HBBMS)

Other threats to City Hospitals were the steady decline in its patient base, which largely had come from the dwindling lower-middle-class neighborhoods surrounding the facility, and a continuing loss of staff physicians.

Many patients who previously had no health insurance and had been compelled to go to City Hospitals for no-cost care were now more likely to be covered by commercial insurance or third-party medical coverage, such as Medicaid and Medicare. They could choose to go elsewhere for care. City Hospitals could not charge the fees that other physicians obtained for services because its physicians were full-time, salaried city employees in a teaching hospital. The city was extremely reluctant to fund new medical positions, upgrade established programs or launch new ones. Staff salaries and benefits, which were controlled by the City Hospitals' department chairs, the dean of the Johns Hopkins School of Medicine, and City Hospitals' board of trustees, ranged from $16,000 to just $43,000, far below the incomes physicians could

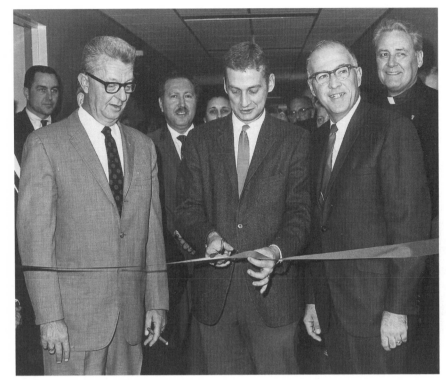

receive from other teaching hospitals in the area. Doctors were leaving; staff vacancies were chronic and critical.[111]

Increasingly frustrated by the low salaries and benefits provided at City Hospitals compared to other medical teaching hospitals in the region, full-time staff decided that the best way to improve their lot was to cease being civil service employees, set up their own nonprofit corporation and sign a contract with the city to provide medical services.

Using as their model the faculty practice plan created at Tufts University Hospital in Boston, a task force under Zieve, obstetrician Frank Kaltreider, radiologist Gaylord Knox, and surgeons Sylvester Sterioff and Gardner Smith obtained permission from the city's board of estimates to hire an accounting firm to explore the feasibility of incorporating as a nonprofit cor-

The Kiwanis Burn Unit at Baltimore City Hospitals was dedicated in November 1968. Thomas J. Krizek, center, performed the ribbon-cutting honors as E. Stephen Farlow (left) president of the Kiwanis Club of Highlandtown, and fellow club members Rev. Bernard P. Scheiner (far right) and Donald E. Hannahs (to Krizek's left) watch. The idea for the special burn unit grew out of a bowling game challenge from Krizek, chief of plastic surgery at the hospital, to fellow Kiwanis member Hannahs to raise funds for burn care. The club, now the Kiwanis Club of East Baltimore, initially gave $20,000 to launch the burn unit; over the next quarter century it would raise more than $1 million for the facility, which evolved into the Baltimore Regional Burn Center and has treated thousands of burn survivors from Maryland, Pennsylvania, Delaware and West Virginia. (HBBMS)

poration. They were convinced that by doing so, they could respond more swiftly to changing medical needs, provide a higher level of care, charge reasonable fees to third-party payers, use the money to enhance their salaries, benefits and research funds, and significantly reduce the city's financial contribution to City Hospitals' operation.[112]

When accountants determined that creating a faculty practice plan at City Hospitals would be financially possible, Zieve and the other physicians got permission

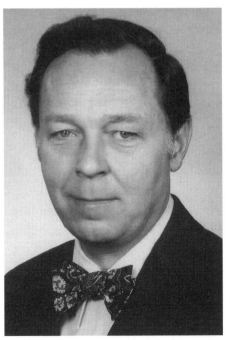

to proceed from the city's board of estimates, composed of Mayor William Donald Schaefer, City Controller Hyman Pressman, and City Council President Walter S. Orlinsky. Concurring in the plan was the dean of the Hopkins School of Medicine, Russell Morgan, to whom most of the City Hospitals physicians reported as full-time members of the school's faculty. The doctors promised city officials they would seek no more in salary support than three-quarters of the $2.2 million the city then was providing for City Hospitals' physicians, or $1.6 million. The rest of their salaries would be covered by the fees they now could charge under the new plan.[113]

Albert Owens, right, began City Hospitals' cancer chemotherapy unit in 1962, creating a program that would provide the foundation for oncology research and treatment at The Johns Hopkins Hospital. (The Alan Mason Chesney Medical Archives of The Johns Hopkins Medical Institutions)

Thus was born Chesapeake Physicians, P.A. (Professional Association), or CPPA, a unique nonprofit corporation formed on September 27, 1972. Initially incorporated as "Kaltreider and Smith," it began operation as "Chesapeake Physicians" (a name suggested by Sterioff) on October 1 with 77 full-time City Hospitals staff members, each of whom paid $1 for a share of stock that offered no dividends (CPPA was nonprofit) but provided each member with a vote. It employed a novel "all-for-one, one-for-all" philosophy that required the various clinical departments to pool their revenues to ensure that no single department had a deficit. Clinical activities and business arrangements were coordinated, and all shared in the successes or failures of the practice. In

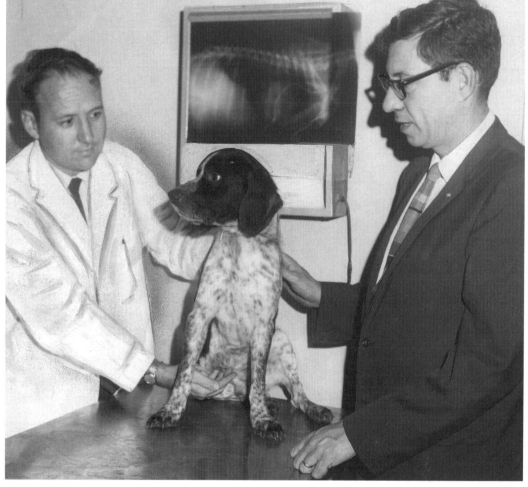

Kenneth B. Lewis, left, chief of cardiology at City Hospitals, and Robert E. Fischell, director of the Space Electric Power System Group at Johns Hopkins' Applied Physics Laboratory (APL), check on "Harry" in November 1969, shortly after Lewis implanted in the dog the first heart pacemaker that could be recharged from outside the body. Developed at the APL as a spinoff of space technology research, the new device ultimately replaced pacemakers that had to be surgically removed from patients to be recharged. The original pacemakers also were bulkier; the APL-developed version was just half an inch thick and weighed only two ounces. (Baltimore News American photo, Special Collections, University of Maryland Libraries. ©The Hearst Corporation.)

time, CPPA became a national model for faculty practice plans in academic medical centers and the subject of a special article in *The New England Journal of Medicine* written by Schmidt, Zieve and Burton D'Lugoff, chief of community medical services.[114] Now virtually every medical school in the country has a faculty practice plan. At least a dozen of them were created after consultation with the founders of CPPA.

CPPA immediately increased the budget for physician and medical staff compensation from the $2.2 million the city had been paying to $4.1 million, with the city responsible only for the $1.6 million it had promised. The remaining $2.5 million came from fees the physicians now could charge third-party payers, including insurance firms and welfare agencies.[115] The city's initial savings of more than half a million dollars grew each year, as its contribution of $1.6 million remained the same but CPPA's budget for medical services rose steadily. Salaries for CPPA members also grew significantly, rising from an average of $30,000 to $45,000 within five years.[116]

At first CPPA was viewed skeptically by some city officials, who saw it primarily as a way for the doctors to get more money for themselves, and with alarm by the city and state medical societies, who worried about "the

Douglas Carroll Jr. (1915-1977) founded the department of rehabilitation and physical medicine in 1957, one of the first units of its kind in the country. He was the first to develop a test for hand function and also concentrated on treating patients with chronic diabetes. A history enthusiast, he wrote a history of medicine in Maryland and a history of Baltimore City Hospitals from which much information in the early portions of this book was drawn. The Carroll Auditorium at Hopkins Bayview is named in his honor. **(HBBMS)**

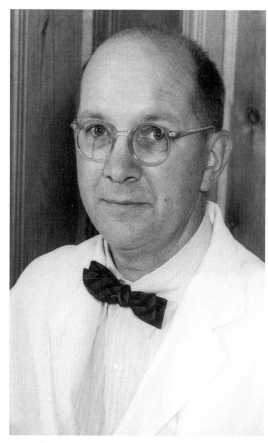

corporate practice of medicine" and the potential competition private practitioners faced from it. But Mayor Schaefer gave the group his support, seeing their model as an innovative way to increase City Hospitals' revenues and reduce the city's financial obligation to the facility.[117]

No longer city employees, the CPPA doctors took control of their professional as well as financial destinies. As members of a nonprofit corporation, their key aim was not to boost their salaries. They wanted financial independence from city government; they wanted to expand their referral base of patients by establishing relationships with independent health maintenance organizations (HMOs) and opening community-based "affiliated community health centers" in the area surrounding the hospital; and they wanted to earn money to pay for more medical research. With the CPPA, they achieved all these goals.[118]

In 1973, City Hospitals celebrated its bicentennial, proudly tracing its lineage back to the Baltimore Almshouse of 1773 and hosting a large community health symposium to mark the anniversary. About 600 people attended the two-day event. By 1973, 90,000 patients were seen annually in City Hospitals' outpatient clinics; 55,000 patients visited the emergency room, and 12,000 patients were admitted.[119] With pardonable pride, City Hospitals boasted about its special burn unit and its innovative, less painful methods for treating severe burns; promoted its infant evacuation system, which used Maryland State Police helicopters to rush critically ill babies in life-support system isolettes to the hospital's neonatal care unit; heralded its large and advanced coronary care center program, which featured Baltimore County Fire Department ambulances equipped with electrocardiogram machines that could radio readings directly to the hospital while racing there with a patient. It cited its cancer chemotherapy research collaboration with The Johns Hopkins Hospital, its crisis unit for handling patients whose severe mental problems prompted suicide attempts, its programs on drug and alcohol abuse; its research in gerontology. City Hospitals' staff of 1,750 included 110 interns and residents.[120]

Representative Paul S. Sarbanes published a tribute to City Hospitals in the *Congressional Record*; Mayor Schaefer issued a proclamation designating November 1973 as "Baltimore City Hospitals Bicentennial Anniversary Month," and the hospital itself published a booklet, "Baltimore City Hospitals: Third Century of Service," that outlined its history and its hopes for a "dynamic future."[121]

Those hopes soon ran up against a range of unremitting problems. Throughout the next crucial decade, City Hospitals would bounce from one financial crisis to another as the city looked desperately for ways to eliminate the red ink from the hospitals' books. City Hospitals had distributed bumper stickers as part of its bicentennial celebration featuring the slogan "Better Community Health." The chronic financial and management problems that subsequently plagued City Hospitals led skeptical and cliché-afflicted local headline writers to title scolding editorials on the hospital's troubles: "Heal Thyself."[122]

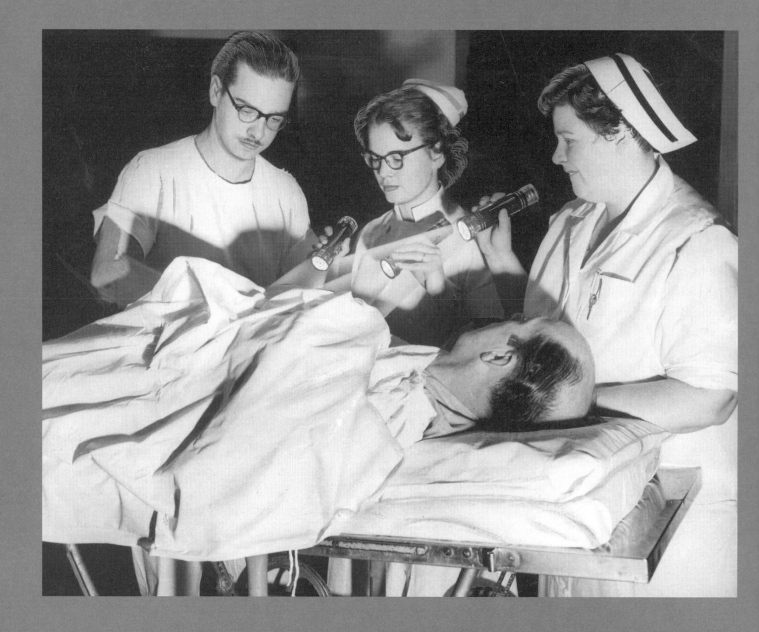

Medicine by flashlight was not uncommon at City Hospitals, where an antiquated power system frequently broke down. Although this photo was taken in 1951, power outage problems persisted into the early 1980s, when Judy Reitz, then director of nursing practices at Hopkins Hospital, visited City Hospitals and found that nurses there kept a large box of more than 100 flashlights handy for emergencies. (Baltimore *News American* photo, Special Collections, University of Maryland Libraries. ©The Hearst Corporation.)

"I Give a 'Damn'"

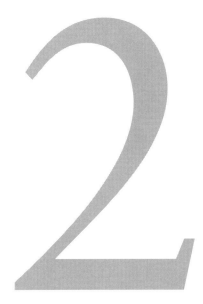

THE CHALLENGES THAT FACED CITY HOSPITALS AS IT ENTERED ITS
third century came as no surprise to its leadership. In a November
1973 article for the *Maryland State Medical Journal* co-authored by
Edmund Beacham, Douglas Carroll and Frederick Hubbard, the
City Hospitals leaders acknowledged that "major changes in social, financial,
and medical practice in the last decade" would require "radical changes in diagnostic methods, treatment, methods of rendering health care, meeting social
problems, and financing medical practice." They recognized that their task
was to provide Baltimore's residents with "the very best medical care using
every innovative financial resource available to assure the lowest cost to the
taxpayers of the City of Baltimore." They conceded that "the financial future
of this institution depends on its recovering a much greater percent of its cost
than it does at present." And they knew accomplishing that goal would require "needed changes [that] promise to be more far reaching than in any
other period in the life of Baltimore City Hospitals."[1]

How far-reaching those changes would turn out to be over the next decade,
they probably had no idea.

By 1973, City Hospitals' annual deficit was nearly $6 million, and no
one in charge seemed quite able to explain precisely why.[2] Key administrative personnel such as the chief financial officer, the operating officer and
the human resources chief were essentially political appointees. Though
several of them had some experience in hospital administration, they had difficulty managing a large, many-faceted institution. "The level of competence

of those senior managers was—I'll use the word 'variable'," Chester Schmidt recalls.[3]

In July 1975, a new IBM computerized billing system was installed in an effort to modernize the institution's fiscal management. It failed miserably and often was out of service for more than half a day at a time. Because the old manual billing system had been scrapped when the computer was installed, the bills for August, September, October and November never were generated or sent out. In late November, *The Sun* published a blistering front-page story on the increasingly desperate situation, headlined "City Hospitals losing millions in fiscal tangle."[4] (The reporter who broke this story was Richard Ben Cramer, who later became a Pulitzer Prize-winning foreign correspondent for the *Philadelphia Inquirer* and author of best-selling books on Joe DiMaggio and on presidential campaigning. Other stories on City Hospitals' financial woes were written by *Evening Sun* reporter Gwen Ifill, now a top journalist for the Public Broadcasting System. Noteworthy physicians were not the only professionals whose apprenticeships brought them to City Hospitals.[5])

Cramer's story described how City Hospitals had not billed for hundreds of thousands of dollars in patient services in the two preceding fiscal years; how the hospital repeatedly missed deadlines for quarterly reports to the state's Health Services Cost Review Commission; how statistics required by state law and for adjustments to Medicare and Medicaid billing were "totally inaccurate"; how outpatient billing was "virtually non-existent"; how boxfuls of computer cards with billing data had been lost; how some physicians practicing at the hospital were permitted to take thousands of dollars' worth of medicines from the hospital pharmacy for free, with the cost of the drugs assigned to a "courtesy account."[6]

Harold Tall, Baltimore's director of information systems, told the City Council's Budget and Finance Committee that he believed City Hospitals' difficulties were repairable, and the malfunctions of the IBM computer's billing operation were "normal start-up problems." Yet when Daniel Paul, the city auditor, presented evidence to the committee that the computers had been out of service for hours on end, newly elected City Councilman Thomas J.S. Waxter Jr. (son of the former city welfare department chief who had been a powerful supporter of City Hospitals in the 1930s) observed that "with the amount of time this system is down, it's almost as if there's no machine there at all."[7]

Mayor William Donald Schaefer ordered the city's Department of Finance, headed by Charles L. Benton Jr., to determine how to reduce the staggering

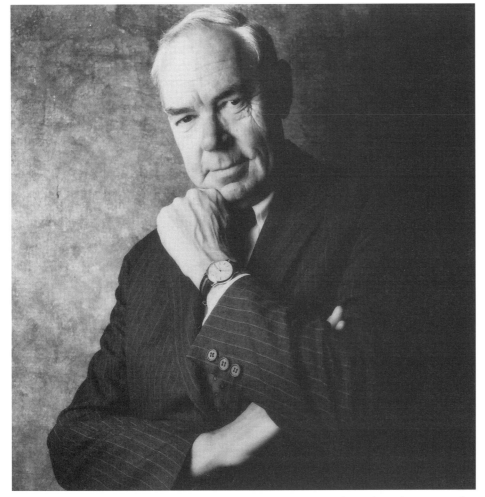

deficit. Benton knew the job would be difficult, contending that the causes for the deficit seemed elusive. "Many hospitals have deficits," he told *The Sun*, "but none of the dimensions found at City Hospitals."[8] By the end of 1975, the deficit was projected to top $8.5 million.[9]

Editorialists decried the "gross mismanagement" at City Hospitals. *The Evening Sun* characterized the hospitals as "a huge money-eating apparatus, a place where they pour taxpayers' money down the drain, even though they don't know exactly where the drain is.

"City Hospitals is a valuable and needed municipal service which should continue. Indeed, there may be compelling reasons why it cannot be a break-even operation and should be subsidized by the taxpayers," *The Evening Sun* continued. "But Baltimoreans have a right to know the cause of the deficit and to expect a sound, tight management to keep the deficit at a minimum. They get neither.... If the current management cannot measure up—as it obviously has not—then Mayor Schaefer... must replace it with competent management."[10]

Within seven months of that editorial admonition, Frederick Hubbard resigned as executive director of City Hospitals in June 1976, ending his

Angry City Hospitals employees wore "I Give a 'Damn'" buttons like the one on the opposite page at a huge 1977 pep rally to refute a city finance department memo claiming that "no one seems to give a damn" at the beleaguered hospital, which was said to be in a state of "anarchy."

William Donald Schaefer, mayor of Baltimore from 1971 to 1987. Early in his tenure he was desperate to get the money-hemorrhaging City Hospitals off the municipal ledger but also to keep it open to serve its Southeast Baltimore community. Later, as governor of Maryland (1987-1995), Schaefer would say that the transfer of City Hospitals to Johns Hopkins was one of the smartest things he did during his 16 years as mayor. (Coutesy C. Fraser Smith)

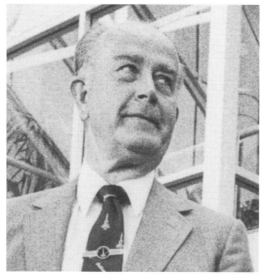

17-year tenure as head of the facility. Although it had urged a change in hospital management, *The Evening Sun* subsequently expressed regret that Hubbard's head was the first to roll. "An unfortunate aspect of Mr. Hubbard's departure is that these financial difficulties tend to obscure his valuable contributions to the development of the hospital over a 17-year period, particularly as a widely recognized center for research into treatment of the aged and the badly burned."

Hubbard was not the last member of City Hospitals' hierarchy to leave the increasingly harried facility. In October 1976, Mayor Schaefer ordered dismissal of most of City Hospitals' financial leadership and told Benton's office to take over day-to-day management there.[11]

A nine-month, nationwide search was conducted to choose Hubbard's successor. In the meantime, lengthy vacancies in the executive director's office—as well as in 13 other top administrative positions at the hospitals—had led to a wave of adverse publicity. "Worker Situation At City Hospitals Reported To Be Nearing 'Anarchy'," blared a front-page banner headline in *The Evening Sun* early in March 1977. "City Hospitals In 'Anarchy,'" proclaimed a headline the same day in the local section of the *News American*.[12]

Both stories cited a memorandum to Mayor Schaefer from his finance director, Benton, forwarding an assessment made by William Schmidt, a management analyst for Benton's department: "One word describes the Hospitals—'ANARCHY'." Schmidt wrote that he had spent at least one day a week at City Hospitals for the preceding seven months and "found a serious breakdown in first-line supervision—no one seems to give a damn."[13]

"From the very outset, by and large, the problems at City Hospitals were not computer problems; it was and remains people problems," Benton told the mayor. Left unsaid in the memo, however, was that City Hospitals' financial managers were, in fact, put in place by Benton's own office. Because of the continuing administrative vacancies at the hospitals, the finance department had taken over their fiscal operations, Benton wrote in his memo. So most of the "first-line supervision" that supposedly had broken down actually was made up of Benton's people.

Both rank-and-file employees and the medical leadership took great exception to the harsh assessment of City Hospitals and rallied to its defense. Philip Zieve, by then chairman of the department of medicine and head of the professional staff committee, denounced the "false allegations in the newspapers" and expressed pride that patient care had not suffered during the long period of fiscal and management turmoil.[14] Paul H. Manner, executive director of the Classified Municipal Employees Association, a union representing some of City Hospitals' workers, called the claim they did not "give a damn" an "absolute lie."

"Apparently Mr. Benton and his henchmen are trying to pass the buck," Manner said. "We suggest they look in the mirror.... The only thing anarchic at City Hospitals is the current department of finance employees who are running the hospital fiscal operation."[15]

Raymond Clark, president of Local 44 of the American Federation of State, County and Municipal Employees, the union representing most blue-collar City Hospitals workers, accused Benton of trying to "cover up his own fiscal blunders at the expense of City Hospitals' employees. I think it's disgraceful and demoralizing and the public should know it."[16]

Hundreds of City Hospitals employees, many wearing buttons proclaiming "I Give a 'Damn'," held a pep rally in its community service center to insist that patient care was not being compromised by the hospitals' financial woes. Burton D'Lugoff, community development director for Chesapeake Physicians, P.A., waved to the crowd and asked a reporter: "Do these people look like anarchists who don't give a damn? We're here to say that if Benton thinks this hospital is approaching anarchy, he is a liar."[17]

D'Lugoff blamed the lengthy administrative vacancies on the city's cumbersome hiring system. "The very same people who are preventing our hiring have turned around and asked, 'Why haven't you filled these vacancies?' Does that make sense?" He and other City Hospitals leaders also were furious that the city adamantly refused to adapt its own computer system, with which it sent out tax and water bills and other invoices, to accommodate an effective hospital billing operation—while publicly proclaiming City Hospitals to be "financially irresponsible."[18]

Mayor Schaefer fumed. He warned that more top-level employees at City Hospitals might be fired, despite the already extensive leadership vacuum there. "There are still people working there who seem to believe they can live with a $3 million deficit," the mayor said.[19]

Schaefer "came out here many times to pound his hands on the table and scream at us for not doing a good enough job," Zieve recalls. "But the reason we weren't doing a good enough job was because the city didn't allow us to do a good enough job, and put a layer of overhead expenses on the hospital which did nothing but direct money to the central city administration and nothing to support the hospital."[20]

Daniel Berger, a veteran editorial writer for *The Evening Sun* (and later *The Sun*), best known for his epigrammatic "Bergerisms," cast his skeptical eye on the City Hospitals situation and assessed it with typical pungency on

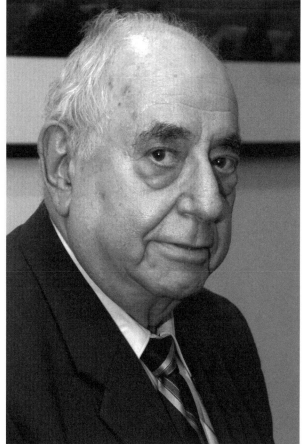

Burton C. D'Lugoff, a founder of Chesapeake Physicians and director of City Hospitals' impressive community medical system, was instrumental in obtaining a $12 million federal grant in 1976 to launch the first health maintenance organization (HMO) in Maryland and became its first medical director. The HMO was named the Metropolitan Baltimore Health Plan but did business as CareFirst. The HMO was acquired by Maryland Blue Cross/Blue Shield in 1991, which began doing business under the name CareFirst Blue Cross/Blue Shield in 1998. (HBBMS)

two separate days: "Pray that City Hospitals is more effective medically than administratively," and "City Hall diagnoses City Hospitals as sick, and vice versa."[21]

Around the country, the 1970s and 1980s were a perilous time for municipal hospitals that treated the urban poor. Many such facilities were faltering. City governments became more and more convinced that they were not equipped financially or administratively to manage or modernize these health care institutions. Philadelphia General Hospital, founded in 1729 and the country's oldest institution in continuous service providing hospital care, was closed in 1977 and eventually demolished. Known affectionately as "Old Blockley" for its location in the former Blockley Township in West Philadelphia, it went out of business because it "no longer met modern standards for a hospital" due to "the need for extensive renovation... to meet the requirements of new fire and other life safety codes...."[22] The venerable St. Louis City Hospital closed in 1985 and left its aging complex, portions of which dated from 1906, to become a decaying eyesore for years.[23]

Schaefer did not want that to happen to Baltimore City Hospitals. Because Medicare and Medicaid had made it possible for poor people to obtain medical treatment at any hospital, the mayor no longer had a strong political reason to keep City Hospitals open for the East Baltimore community in which it was located and which long had been a political stronghold for him. Yet, though he repeatedly threatened to close the hospital, he continued looking for ways to keep it open.[24]

Within two weeks of the "anarchy" stories, the mayor filled the top slot at City Hospitals by picking George Havercheck, a former vice president of Buffalo General Hospital, to be the new executive director of the facility. "I have met with Mr. Havercheck personally, and I am impressed by his forthrightness, his drive and his obvious ability to do the job," Schaefer told the press in mid-March 1977.

"Mr. Havercheck has a particularly strong background in fiscal affairs. As a result of this, I am confident that Mr. Havercheck, working with the appropriate city agencies, will be successful in putting the hospital on a firm financial footing."[25] The mayor added that he had assured Havercheck, "I have no intention of closing City Hospitals and... I have no intention of turning it over to the state."

Despite its financial woes, City Hospitals had a number of attractive assets, among them the increasingly powerful and effective Chesapeake Physicians Professional Association. By 1977, five years after its founding, CPPA's membership had grown from 68 to 88 physicians. It had expanded its referral base by participating in the creation of three health maintenance organizations (HMOs), opening a comprehensive ambulatory care facility, the $1.1 million

Greater Dundalk Medical Center, and becoming involved in the development of four more health care outreach centers. CPPA also won a significant contract to provide primary and specialty care for more than 2,000 inmates in the Baltimore City Jail. The Robert Wood Johnson Foundation awarded it a $2.85 million grant to establish three more walk-in clinics.[26] "We're not guaranteed our business at all," the CPPA's president, Chester Schmidt, told *The Evening Sun* in 1978. "We have to go out and drum up business."[27]

Burton D'Lugoff did the lion's share of the drumming. He oversaw the development of City Hospitals' impressive community medical system and was instrumental in obtaining a $12 million federal grant in 1976 to launch the first health maintenance organization (HMO) based in Maryland, the Metropolitan Baltimore Health Plan, which did business under the name CareFirst.[28] (CareFirst was acquired by Maryland Blue Cross/Blue Shield in 1991, and Blue Cross subsequently adopted the CareFirst name for all of its mid-Atlantic managed care operations. By 2003, CareFirst had morphed into a mammoth, independent, nonprofit holding company providing health care services to nearly 3.2 million members in Maryland, Delaware, the District of Columbia and portions of Virginia.)[29]

In 1977, D'Lugoff became the first medical director of the original CareFirst and almost simultaneously launched a state-mandated HMO, the Chesapeake Health Plan, and a third CPPA-developed HMO, the Baltimore Medical System, created in conjunction with Blue Cross.[30] He found a ready market for their services in Southeast Baltimore's still-thriving, heavily unionized blue-collar community. "We had a very strong assist from the union leadership" of the local United Steelworkers, United Auto Workers and other unions representing electrical and warehouse workers, D'Lugoff recalls. Baltimore "was still an

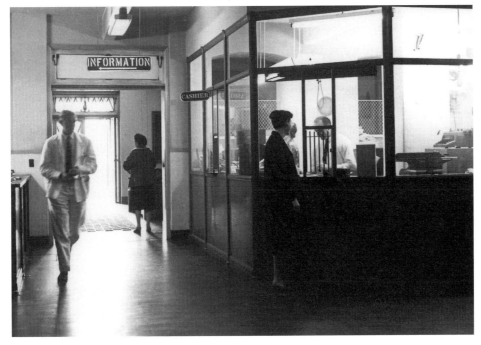

The check-in counter at the **City Hospitals' A Building,** the acute care facility, as it looked in the late 1960s and early 1970s. (HBBMS)

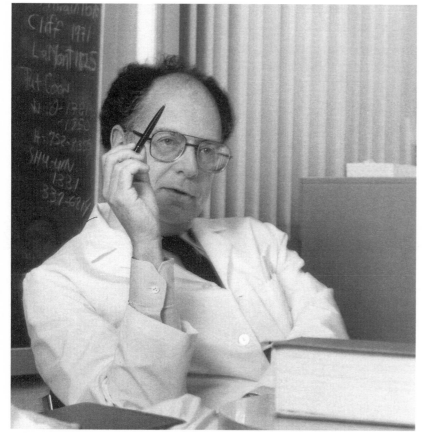

Philip Zieve joined the staff of City Hospitals in 1964 and became an internationally recognized hematologist, as well as chairman of the Department of Medicine and chief of the professional staff for more than 25 years. Among the founders of Chesapeake Physicians Professional Association, he and Chester Schmidt worked behind the scenes to persuade Baltimore City and Hopkins Hospital to reach an agreement that would save City Hospitals. (HBBMS)

industrial giant" in the mid-1970s, D'Lugoff notes, with Bethlehem Steel "going full tilt," keeping up to 100,000 employees on its mid-Atlantic payroll—a heavy concentration of them in its landmark Sparrow's Point facility in Baltimore.[31]

D'Lugoff and his associates would hold community sessions and meetings in the plants to promote CareFirst's services, for which City Hospitals was the exclusive medical provider. The CPPA had opened attractive community medical centers on North Point Boulevard, on Dundalk Avenue (in a converted funeral parlor, much to the grim amusement of the residents) and elsewhere, all of them bearing the CareFirst logo. HMOs at the time were considered socially advanced (some detractors called them "communistic," D'Lugoff recalls), and the lower, prepaid medical costs they offered were appreciated both by the union members and their employers.[32]

In promoting CareFirst, Chesapeake Health and Baltimore Medical, D'Lugoff stressed the new, attractive, semi-private community practice centers in which union members would be receiving 95 percent of their medical care, not the contracts' fine print, which said they would have to go to City Hospitals if they required hospitalization. If that issue was raised at a meeting, the CPPA representative would insist that the old place had undergone considerable refurbishment—there were telephones and televisions in the rooms now, as well as other amenities—and in short order, the CPPA was bringing a steady flow of new patients to City Hospitals.[33] In 1977, the first year of Care-First's operation, CPPA reported revenues of $7,634,000.

By 1980, CPPA's revenues would nearly double to $14,202,876. Its staff consisted of 139 full-time professionals, 131 of them physicians, distributed through nine of City Hospitals' departments: anesthesia, medicine, neurology, obstetrics and gynecology, pathology, psychiatry, radiology, dermatology and surgery. Its members obtained $2.9 million in research grants that year. And as part of City Hospitals' long-standing association with the Johns Hopkins School of Medicine, all of the CPPA physicians had faculty appointments at Hopkins, as had previous City Hospitals doctors.[34]

The achievements of the CPPA notwithstanding, Havercheck could not stem the flow of red ink or the onslaught of black headlines compounding and proclaiming the problems at City Hospitals. He was unable to fix the hospitals' chaotic billing procedures, and the deficits continued to mount. He lasted just three and a half years on the job. The mayor, increasingly frustrated, removed him from office in October 1981 and swiftly replaced him with A. Yvonne Russell, the head of the U.S. Public Health Service Hospital in Boston. She would remain a scant seven months.[35]

As much as he was determined to keep City Hospitals open to serve the health care needs of Southeast Baltimore, Schaefer also was desperately seeking to get Baltimore City out of the hospital business. He hoped to hand City Hospitals' management over to the state (abandoning his earlier pledge not to do so) or turn it into a nonprofit, public-interest corporation, thereby wiping its whopping deficits off the city's ledger.[36]

In 1980, Baltimore's voters approved a change in the City Charter, recommended by a Schaefer-appointed commission, that would transform City Hospitals into a public-interest corporation. The City Council had not passed legislation to permit this by the time Havercheck was replaced by Russell, but the mayor successfully pushed for creation of the new hospital corporation, The Medical Center of Baltimore, Inc. It was to be governed by a 15-member board appointed by the mayor, and aim to attract individual doctors and their patients to the hospital, which then was operating at a pale 74 percent of capacity.[37]

The mayor telephoned his old friend and political ally, Governor Marvin Mandel. "I said, 'Marvin, we want you to take City Hospitals,'" Schaefer recalled years later. "He said, 'You're my friend, Don, and I hope you'll continue to be, but we're not taking City Hospitals under any circumstances!'"[38]

Spurned by the state, Schaefer started looking for other ways to unload City Hospitals while keeping it open. The city let it be known it would entertain bids from for-profit health care companies to take over operation of City Hospitals. Interest was shown by such firms as the Hospital Corporation of America (HCA), the world's largest owner of hospitals, operating 349 facilities with a combined total of more than 49,000 beds; and American Medical International (AMI), then the second largest owner of hospitals in the world.[39]

Closely watching the developments at City Hospitals was Robert Heyssel, then executive vice president and soon to be president of The Johns Hopkins Hospital. Heyssel was an extraordinarily savvy observer of the health care field nationwide. Against the prevailing consensus of many administrators of major hospitals, he had the foresight to envision the continued growth of managed care companies, which would put significant pressure on nonprofit hospitals such as Hopkins. He believed that Hopkins needed to expand in order to counteract the potential competition, and he did not want to see a for-profit firm taking over City Hospitals.[40]

In the fall of 1981, Heyssel and Edward Halle, Hopkins Hospital's senior

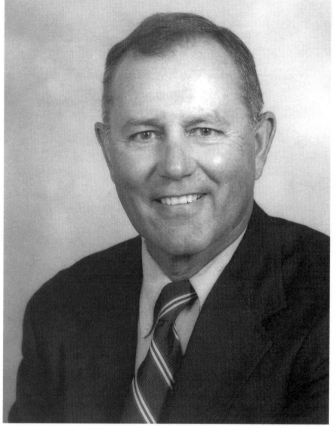

Chester W. Schmidt Jr. has been chief of the Department of Psychiatry since 1972. He was among the founders of the Chesapeake Physicians practice group, later Hopkins Bayview Physicians, and served as its president for nearly a quarter century. Renowned in his field for his extensive contributions to the literature, particularly the study of suicide, he has overseen an immensely beneficial expansion of Hopkins Bayview's community psychiatric services, which now handle nearly 114,000 visits annually. (HBBMS)

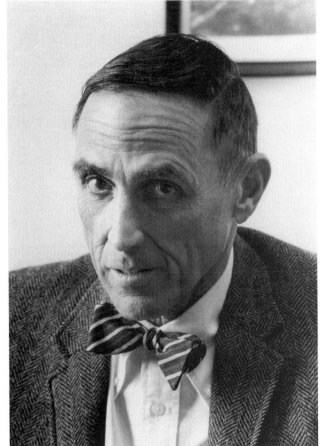

Edward Halle, senior vice president for administration of The Johns Hopkins Hospital during Robert Heyssel's tenure as president. He was among the first to suggest that the improvement in City Hospitals' finances after a year of Hopkins' management in 1982-83 warranted its acquisition. He became Hopkins' chief negotiator during the lengthy wrangling with city officials over the terms for acquiring City Hospitals. (The Alan Mason Chesney Medical Archives of The Johns Hopkins Medical Institutions)

vice president for administration, were having lunch with several other hospital officials in the Sheraton motel that then was across Broadway from their offices in Hopkins' famous domed administration building. "We were talking about the fact that these for-profits were interested in coming to town, and Heyssel, in particular, didn't think that was a good idea... and maybe we ought to look into it," Halle recalls.[41]

In September 1981, *The Sun* reported that The Johns Hopkins Hospital was expressing an interest in taking over management of City Hospitals in 1982. Elaine Freeman, the chief spokesperson for Hopkins, confirmed for the paper that the hospital was "making a feasibility study" to determine if it wanted to offer a bid to manage City Hospitals.[42]

Among those participating in the feasibility study was Judy Reitz, who had been hired as director of nursing practices at The Johns Hopkins Hospital only two months before. Heyssel had asked her boss, Martha Sacci, vice president for nursing at the hospital, to go out to City Hospitals to assess its nursing and long-term care programs. Sacci, evidently considering Heyssel's request a relatively low priority, sent her young assistant instead.[43]

Reitz spent the week of September 10 through September 18 at City Hospitals, and what she found there both stunned and impressed her. "I had never seen conditions of patient care like that in my entire career," she recalls. The nursing facilities conveyed a "nearly World War II kind of vintage atmosphere." Due to the aging electrical system, power outages were so frequent that the nurses kept a box of more than 100 flashlights handy for emergencies—and checked the batteries regularly.[44]

Despite the "amazingly poor physical facilities," the substandard wages, the difficulties of recruiting full-time nurses and the resulting need to use temporary agency employees, what impressed Reitz most was the "huge commitment to care," in both the nursing department and the acute care hospital. Her report to Sacci stressed "the rich potential" at City Hospitals.[45]

After *The Sun* broke the story about Hopkins' tentative "feasibility" inquiries, Albert M. Antlitz, the newly appointed chairman of the soon-to-be-installed board of the Medical Center of Baltimore (the new official name for City Hospitals) told the paper that it was "premature" to discuss Hopkins' assumption of management, but that the board would be "receptive" to any Hopkins proposal.[46]

Spurring Heyssel's interest in City Hospitals was an ongoing lobbying campaign undertaken by Philip Zieve and Chester Schmidt, who sought to convince him that Hopkins should take over the besieged but promising institution.

"We had been to Bob Heyssel, several of us, a number of times, to ask whether Hopkins would not be favored by taking over," Zieve recalls. "He was interested in it, but was never sure he could get it past his board."[47]

"I can't tell you the hours that we spent lobbying the mayor on one side and Bob Heyssel on the other—first to get Hopkins involved, which we did, and then to complete the deal," Schmidt says. Heyssel "was very reticent about this whole thing, and it took a lot of jawboning on our part to help him see the wisdom of his final decision."[48]

Shortly before his death in 2001, Heyssel recalled: "Hopkins had a huge stake in the continuance of City Hospitals. The Chesapeake Physicians group there were all [Hopkins] faculty members... and they... [were] quite distinguished.... And a major amount of teaching went on there, as well as research." Apart from the CPPA and the Hopkins medical students who were taught at City Hospitals, Heyssel noted that the region's only burn unit was there; the National Institute of Aging had its major research facility there. He had also heard that the federal government's research program on drugs and drug abuse, then located in Kentucky, would move to City Hospitals if Hopkins took over there.

"So there were a lot of reasons for Hopkins to be interested in an arrangement that either allowed us to manage or outright own City Hospitals," Heyssel recalled.[49] A tall, blunt-spoken Missouri native, Heyssel became convinced he had to cut off prospective competitors at the pass.[50]

One of the for-profit companies approached Heyssel and asked him if Hopkins would be interested in running City Hospitals if the firm acquired it. Heyssel rejected the company's offer and determined to undercut its bid should it attempt to take over on Eastern Avenue. He approached Schaefer and told him that Hopkins would be interested in managing City Hospitals for nothing, simply at cost, since Hopkins was not looking to make money off the facility. By tendering this offer, he hoped to prevent any for-profit company from moving into Hopkins' territory.[51] Heyssel and the Hopkins medical school dean, Richard Ross, had decided that if Hopkins could manage City Hospitals for a trial period and start reducing its staggering deficits, perhaps Hopkins might consider taking it over permanently.

In April 1982, Schaefer announced that he had suggested that Hopkins, rather than a for-profit health care company, manage the hospital.[52] The mayor recognized that Baltimore City had a duty to the people in its blue-collar southeast section that was more important than maximizing the cash that might come from selling City Hospitals to a for-profit health care company. He had become convinced that only Hopkins would continue providing medical services to the low-income and indigent residents of that area, regardless of their ability to pay.[53] (Hopkins Hospital always had accepted charity cases, and in the early 1980s it actually had more nonpaying patients than City Hospitals.)[54]

At the same time the Schaefer administration invited Hopkins to submit a proposal to assume management of City Hospitals, it also asked discreetly if Hopkins wanted to acquire the entire facility outright. Heyssel and Ross decided they would allow themselves to be wooed and set about persuading the Hopkins Hospital trustees that acquisition of City Hospitals merited consideration.[55]

At an executive session of the Hopkins Hospital's board of trustees on May 4, 1982, Steven Muller, president of the university and hospital, reported that the Joint Committee of Trustees had approved in principle a strategic plan to create a corporation to own and operate joint ventures for the institutions. Among those ventures, Heyssel and Ross explained, might be City Hospitals. Both Heyssel and Ross stressed that Hopkins needed to ensure the permanent access of its medical house staff to the diverse mix of cases available for training purposes at City Hospitals, and that with the expansion of specialty care to community hospitals, Hopkins had to view its market now as a competitive one. City Hospitals could provide an important competitive edge.[56]

Persuaded by Heyssel and Ross' presentation, the Hopkins Hospital board of trustees gave the go-ahead to begin formal negotiations for acquiring City Hospitals, noting in a prepared statement that such a venture "would represent a major step for both the city and Hopkins," and therefore required "adequate investigation and deliberation on both sides."[57]

Heyssel planned to drive a tough bargain. Essential requirements for such a deal, he told the board of trustees, would include absolving Hopkins from any of City Hospitals' financial liabilities; acquiring all of City Hospitals' real estate and projects at no cost; provision of sufficient working capital from the city; and a five-year reversion clause giving Hopkins the option of returning City Hospitals to the city if it proved to be a financial sinkhole.[58]

Once it was announced that Hopkins Hospital's board of trustees had agreed to formal bargaining for a takeover of City Hospitals, Benton revealed that he and his deputy, Harold Tall, had quietly participated in "exploratory... fact-finding" talks with Hopkins about managing City Hospitals as early as March 1982.[59] This revelation evidently surprised some members of City Hospitals' "transition" board of trustees, who had been authorized to convert it into a private, nonprofit community hospital, and to City Hospitals' executive director, Russell, who knew little of what was going on behind the scenes. Frustrated by what she later called "the bureaucracy of the City of Baltimore," Russell abruptly quit in July 1982. She told the press that she had been "left in the dark for the last three-and-a-half to four months," and that both she and her efforts to plan for City Hospitals' conversion to a nonprofit hospital had been "left in limbo... during the time negotiations have been going on with Hopkins.... I'm not told anything."[60] Accepting a position as an assistant to the president of the University of Texas' medical branch in Galveston, Russell said she would leave City Hospitals by September 1.[61]

Broadway Medical Management Corporation—the subsidiary of Hopkins that Heyssel earlier had urged be created to oversee such ventures as the marketing of the new Johns Hopkins Health Plan, a managed care company—won the City Hospitals' management contract in August 1982, when the city's board of estimates approved its proposal.[62]

To fill the vacancy created by Russell's sudden resignation, Heyssel quickly settled on a 34-year-old protégé of his, Ronald R. Peterson, who had begun work at Hopkins Hospital as an administrative resident in 1973 and rapidly assumed managerial positions of increasing importance with marked success.

Born in New Brunswick, New Jersey, Peterson entered The Johns Hopkins University as a freshman in 1966, hoping to pursue a career as a physician. During his undergraduate years, however, his father became gravely ill, and Peterson could see that medical school would "not be in the cards" for him, given his family's financial situation. After graduating from Hopkins in 1970, he became a biology teacher at the Mergenthaler Vocational-Technical High School in Baltimore and taught adult education courses at night. With a wife and two small children, he supplemented his income by working part-time as a manager for a Baltimore catering firm.

Peterson never lost his interest in medicine, however, and when a friend suggested he explore The George Washington University's

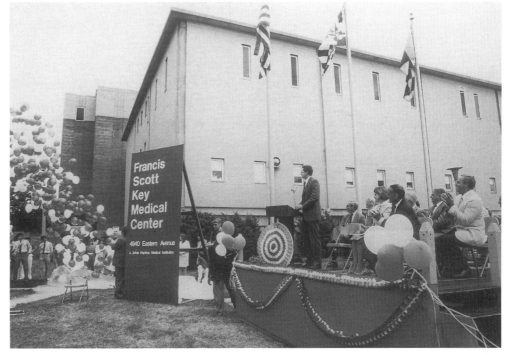

A bevy of balloons signaled the official affiliation of The Johns Hopkins Hospital and the Francis Scott Key Medical Center on July 2, 1984. Ronald R. Peterson, FSKMC's president, at the podium, watches the unveiling of the facility's new name sign by William Ward, vice president for operations, as officials from Baltimore and Hopkins look on. (HBBMS)

master's degree in hospital administration, he followed that advice, entered the program and obtained his degree in 1973. He leapt at the opportunity to do his administrative residency at Hopkins, where he soon drew Heyssel's attention as a promising young administrator.

As administrator of the 75-bed Henry Phipps Psychiatric Clinic from 1974 to 1975, Peterson reduced its annual rate of unit cost increase from 12 percent to 5 percent. From 1975 to 1978, he developed and administered the Hopkins Cost Improvement Program, which became nationally famous as it achieved $3 million in savings for the hospital over Peterson's three-year tenure. When he took over administration of Hopkins' 200-bed Children's Medical and Surgical Center, he maximized revenues by reorganizing its outpatient services, which handled 110,000 visits annually, and introduced a new billing service that substantially increased professional fee receipts. When Heyssel founded

Broadway Medical Management and became its president, he named Peterson its vice president. A headline in *The Evening Sun* dubbed Peterson "a fiscal surgeon." Heyssel decided he was just the man to cure City Hospitals' ills.

"He caught our attention with his energy, his good judgment, as a very young man," Heyssel recalled years later. "He did a remarkably good job in all these [previous] roles, and so when we needed someone to go down and manage City Hospitals for a year, 'til we could see whether we thought we could really acquire it, he was really one of the obvious choices."[63]

Peterson was named executive director of City Hospitals and took over there on September 13, 1982. He asked two other young Hopkins administrators to accompany him to Eastern Avenue: William Ward, 38, who had been associate administrator of the Johns Hopkins Oncology Center, as chief operating officer; and 36-year-old Kenneth Grabill, an associate director of operations, planning and budgets at the Hopkins Hospital, as chief financial officer.

Grabill, born in Frederick, Maryland, had a hardscrabble upbringing. His father, a dairy farmer turned carpenter, died when he was 13, leaving his mother to eke out a living cleaning houses and babysitting. From the age of 14, Grabill supplemented their income by working at a series of jobs while going to school. He obtained a degree in accounting from the University of Baltimore, landed positions as an accountant for the Baltimore Orioles and on the auditing staff of the Coopers & Lybrand accounting firm, then began his health services career at Hopkins in 1974. His up-by-his-own-bootstraps background proved "very helpful to me in coming here to work at Baltimore City Hospitals, the former welfare hospital," Grabill says. Although he is "very conservative" in financial matters, "boy, do I have sensitive feelings about people who are disadvantaged," he notes. He has been there.[64]

Ward, born in Brooklyn, New York, earned his undergraduate degree from Mt. St. Mary's College and his M.B.A. from Loyola College. He entered the Air Force during the Vietnam War and served in Alaska, Kansas, Texas and Indiana, primarily in public affairs work. He was a TV and radio reporter—"the voice of the Alaskan Air Command"—for a year and also edited a weekly newspaper. After his military service, Ward and his wife, a Baltimorean whom he had met while in college, decided to settle in her home town. He held accounting jobs at Good Samaritan Hospital and elsewhere before coming to the Hopkins oncology center in 1976.[65]

Peterson, Ward and Grabill formed the three-man team that would tackle the job of turning around City Hospitals while simultaneously making an in-depth analysis of whether it was feasible for Hopkins to acquire the facility. Peterson then would report on their efforts and the results to the Joint Policy Committee of Hopkins trustees. In taking these new positions, all three men realized, Ward recalls, that "there was no jumping out of the airplane and getting back in." If Hopkins decided not to acquire City Hospitals or continue managing it, "there was no guarantee we could get our old jobs back," although each man was given written assurance that "every effort would be made" to find him a position at Hopkins if the City Hospitals experiment failed.

Grabill recalls walking with Peterson past the Phipps building at Hopkins late one night, having put in another horrifically long day at both City Hospitals and Hopkins, and wondering aloud, "Are these guys, Heyssel and company, going to save any space for us when this fails? Where are we going to have offices?" With gallows humor, Peterson pointed down to a lighted basement window. "They're probably going to put us in the basement here at Phipps," he said.[66]

Although there was a risk in going to City Hospitals, Ward says, there also was the opportunity to accomplish great things. "I don't think I ever for a moment doubted that we could do it."[67] Grabill recalls that the move to City Hospitals "was *very scary,* although at the same time, very rewarding, because whatever you did here made a difference.... There was so much to be fixed."[68]

When he arrived at City Hospitals, Peterson says, he felt as if he were taking a journey back in time. Many of the physical facilities were extremely old; the Mason F. Lord Building, albeit periodically updated, had been built in 1866. Infrastructure was rickety or worse. His first day on the job, Peterson discovered that the electrical system had no functioning emergency generator—and the Joint Commission on the Accreditation of Healthcare Organizations was scheduled to arrive the following week for its regular inspection. Peterson promptly rented an emergency generator, had it placed on a truck, and hooked it up to the main power plant. He also found many patient rooms were still multiple-occupancy, and the patient accounting system was in shambles. He walked into one room and discovered piles of shoeboxes filled to overflowing with bills that had not been sent.[69]

Yet Peterson also saw enormous potential for turning the situation around, fixing the financial mess, erasing the chronic deficits and putting City Hospitals back in the black. The key was that "the city did not really understand the *business* of contemporary medicine," which Peterson and his team understood intimately. "So we saw tremendous opportunities to improve the financial performance of the hospital," he recalls.[70]

He was especially impressed with Chesapeake Physicians and its leadership. "The presence of that well-organized, well-credentialed physicians' group was really what made us say, 'Yes, this is going forward,'" Peterson says. He soon developed a close working relationship with Zieve, Schmidt and Gardner Smith, chairman of the surgery department.

Also on the scene was Walter Schneckenberger, a former long-time chief financial officer at Baltimore's Sinai Hospital, who earlier had been hired as a consultant by the city to help manage City Hospitals. Although, as Grabill notes, Schneckenberger was basically Baltimore's "control on the scene, spy

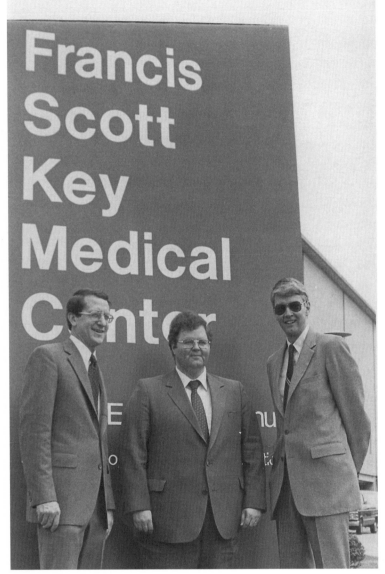

The close collaboration between a team of young Hopkins Hospital administrators, led by (left to right) **Ronald R. Peterson, Kenneth Grabill** and **William Ward**, shown here in 1984, and the leadership of City Hospitals' physicians' practice group led to the financial turnaround of the institution and its transformation into the Francis Scott Key Medical Center and ultimately Johns Hopkins Bayview Medical Center. (HBBMS)

and protector of the interests of the city," he proved to be "an absolute joy" for Grabill to work with in trying to unravel City Hospitals' tangled financial operations. "He had a fabulous knowledge and super integrity," Grabill says.[71]

Peterson quickly improved the hospital's collection rate by installing a new billing system and training the accounts receivable staff in good business practices, including following up on unpaid bills—something that simply never had been done there before.[72] He and his staff improved cost controls and increased productivity levels by introducing proper supervision and incentives for personnel to do their work and measure their accomplishments.[73]

"They rode herd on the existing personnel. Those who didn't cut it were moved on, and they brought additional talent into the claims and billing offices," Schmidt recalls. "What they did was do the basic fundamentals of hospital administration and finance. They had a massive clean-up job, and then they put in place systems that were reliable. So for the first time, maybe ever, the hospital had reliable financial systems producing clean claims and getting bills out in a timely fashion."[74]

The inefficient billing computer system that had led to such terrible publicity in 1975 still was in place—and still not working right. Bills still were being prepared manually by compiling paper slips for service charges that then were fed haphazardly into the computer, which had never been correctly programmed to handle the accounts of a major acute-care hospital. Grabill and Schneckenberger worked together to reinstall the computer system so it would accurately register and admit patients, capture billing and demographic information, and tote up a bill for services provided. They then retrained or replaced billing and patient registration personnel to ensure that the technology was used properly. Significant sums in open receivables were also recovered when methodical billing and collection practices were implemented.[75]

In addition, the Peterson team greatly improved City Hospitals' inadequate procedures for ensuring that self-paid, no-pay and indigent patients qualified for Medicaid. Other hospitals in the city, including Hopkins, already were doing this. By gathering data from poor patients and taking the initiative to complete Medicaid applications for them, City Hospitals at last received millions of dollars in state Medicaid funds to cover hospital bills that previously had gone unpaid.[76]

Peterson's swift success in starting to set City Hospitals' financial house in order enabled him and his colleagues to deal effectively with the state's Health Services Cost Review Commission (HSCRC), an agency City Hospitals' previous municipal administrators had found daunting in the extreme.

The HSCRC sets rates for hospitals by comparing their services with those offered by "peer group" facilities in the area. In December 1982, Grabill and Schneckenberger put together an "impeccable" case to demonstrate to the HSCRC that "based on the service characteristics" of the patients treated at City Hospitals, the price structure that the HSCRC had set for it was "understated by 23 percent," Grabill recalls. His efforts to explain this to the city finance officials who long before should have corrected this error was met with glazed eyes.[77] The HSCRC promptly authorized City Hospitals to raise its rates by 23 percent.

"I got the draft of the rate order that empowered the hospital to do this charge-up... on a day when Peterson was doing all sorts of important things," Grabill recalls. When he showed it to Peterson, "Ron said, 'Stop all else.' He took me in his car to the offices of the Health Services Cost Review Commission to get the final rate order in hand. When we had the 23 percent [increase]... we knew... we were going to achieve a financial turnaround. It sealed the deal for success."[78] (Three years later, they would learn that what the HSCRC could give, it also could take away or reduce. The challenge to reverse City Hospitals' decline was far from finished.)

By demonstrating a command of City Hospitals' finances that their predecessors had never been able to display, the Peterson team—aided by support from Hopkins—substantially improved City Hospitals' total revenues, cutting dramatically into the deficit.

"Ron went out there and within a year had cut the operating loss from $7 million to $1 million," Heyssel recalled, "and I told him to stop, because I said, 'Ron, you're going to make it valuable to the city.'"[79]

In February 1983, Peterson presented a report to the joint committee of Hopkins Hospital and University trustees, detailing the financial turnaround on Eastern Avenue and proposing that Hopkins acquire the facility. He had determined that City Hospitals could break even financially but needed a multimillion-dollar renovation and new construction program over the long haul.[80] Heyssel remained cautious. He had genuine concern about whether Hopkins wanted to take over a hospital that had a crumbling plant, an essentially impoverished clientele—and a reputation of having gone downhill for years.[81]

As Peterson was preparing his report to the trustees, Ed Halle decided the improved financial circumstances at City Hospitals was so impressive that Hopkins should acquire it. He suggested to Heyssel that they approach Walter Sondheim, a former president of the city school board, a long-time advisor to city mayors and a good friend of Halle's, and have him "tell the mayor to sell us City Hospitals for a dollar."

Heyssel did not jump at the idea, Halle recalls. "He kind of grunted and went on with whatever he was doing, and I went back to my office in the administration building—and when I walked in, Walter Sondheim was sitting at my desk, using my phone!"

This serendipitous encounter stemmed from Halle's arrangement for a free parking space near his office for Sondheim, who, though he was not a physician, frequently visited the hospital as a community member of the board that reviewed proposals for human research at Hopkins. That day, Sondheim had dropped by to say hello to his friend Halle and, in his absence, sat down to use his telephone.

"So I told him what I just had said to Bob Heyssel... , and he said, 'Well, I'm going to see the mayor in a few minutes. I won't be able to talk to him about it today, but I will see him again tomorrow.'" Sondheim then left Halle's office, but promptly the next afternoon, around 5 p.m., he called.

"He said, 'Were you serious in what you said yesterday?' And I said, 'I don't know; Bob Heyssel's sitting right here, let me ask him.' I said, "Bob, Walter wants to know if I was serious yesterday.' He said, 'Yeah, you were serious.' So I said, 'Walter, Bob says I was serious.' He said, 'O.K.'," Halle recalls.

Sondheim met with Mayor Schaefer that evening. "He told me not to lose any time in getting started on this," recalls Sondheim, now 95 years old and still actively engaged in city affairs. "He only had to hear [Halle's proposal] for five minutes before he was ready to go."[82]

The next morning, the mayor created a committee to negotiate for what originally was to be a sale of City Hospitals to Hopkins for a dollar. Ultimately it turned out to be an agreement by which the city paid Hopkins millions to take it over.[83]

On March 10, 1983, following another presentation by Peterson to the joint committee of university and hospital trustees of his analysis of the advantages of acquiring City Hospitals, the combined trustees unanimously approved initiation of formal negotiations for its takeover.[84]

The bargaining for this extraordinary deal actually would continue, on and off, for more than a year. Benton and his deputy, Harold Tall, were canny negotiators, but in Heyssel, Ed Halle, Hopkins Hospital chief financial officer Irvin Kues, Peterson and Grabill, they had met their match.[85] The city, always financially strapped, wanted to get as much money as it could for City Hospitals' facilities and the 134 acres of land surrounding them—one of the largest parcels of relatively undeveloped real estate in the city. Hopkins, leery of assuming responsibility for a run-down hospital complex that had lost millions of dollars over the years, wanted to minimize its risks. Heyssel felt Hopkins would take on "a good deal of risk and heavy potential liability" if an acquired City Hospitals turned out to be an albatross.[86] He was determined to stick to the essential elements for an acquisition deal that he had outlined to Hopkins Hospital's board of trustees in May of 1982.

Brought in to help broker the deal were two municipal gray eminences, Sondheim and George McGowan, president of Baltimore Gas and Electric Co. and a member of the board of trustees then overseeing City Hospitals.[87] Also taking part in the negotiations were attorneys Barry Rosen, serving as outside counsel to the city, and Richard Tillman, working on behalf of Hopkins. In the end, thanks to Heyssel, Halle, Kues, Peterson and Grabill, Hopkins got City Hospitals and its land for better than nothing. And Schaefer, Benton and Tall were delighted with the outcome. At last the multimillion-dollar deficits from City Hospitals were wiped off Baltimore's books.[88]

As the city's primary negotiator, Benton brought an unusual combination of qualities to the bargaining table. Laconic in speech, shrewd and innovative in fiscal matters, he also was intensely religious. "You would go into his conference area, and all of the Bibles would be lined up," Peterson recalls. "We didn't actually have to pray before each meeting, but it felt like it." Once, before other members of the negotiating team had arrived in Benton's office, Grabill found himself alone with the city's financial chief. Benton slipped a small pamphlet across the table to him. Its title: "Can You Prove There Is No Hell?" Grabill needed no convincing. "Each of those meetings felt like hell," he now says, laughing.[89]

Benton's initial negotiating gambit was to put an estimated value of $100 million on the City Hospitals land and facilities—many of which were, in Heyssel's view, good only for tearing down. And, hewing to the quirk of municipal accounting by which Baltimore city viewed City Hospitals' millions in accounts receivable as an asset rather than a bad debt, Benton added these into the equation in calculating the institution's worth.[90]

"I think at the first meeting, Benton said, 'Well, how much is Hopkins going to pay us for City Hospitals?' We all knew each other, and I started to laugh," Sondheim recalls with a grin. "And Benton wondered why I laughed. And I said, you all are too young to have been O. Henry fans, but this idea [of Hopkins paying to take over City Hospitals] reminds me of 'The Ransom of Red Chief'," the classic story of two grifters who unwittingly kidnap a horrible brat whose parents are only too glad to see him go. The kidnappers eventually pay the parents to take the kid back.[91]

Often, when a Hopkins official cited a major deficiency in City Hospitals' facilities, Benton would seek to downplay the problem or even turn it into an asset. Once Halle pointed out to Benton that one of the City Hospitals buildings had a heating and air conditioning system that was more than 40 years old. "I quipped that it must be a pretty darn good system if it lasted that long, and I wouldn't recommend getting rid of it," Benton recalled years later, with a chuckle.[92]

Negotiations dragged on. Although Heyssel and Halle believed Hopkins would be protecting itself from pending competition if it acquired City

Hospitals, other members of the Hopkins medical leadership were not persuaded that such a threat was imminent. "Not all of the Hopkins players were on the same song sheet," Peterson recalls, and issues about the acquisition effort had to be ironed out among them, even as the negotiations with the city continued. For its part, the city's bargaining team kept pushing for Hopkins to pay "major dollars" to acquire the acreage and buildings. Hopkins' negotiators had to convince the city that Hopkins should not have to pay anything in return for agreeing to maintain the uncompensated care tradition at City Hospitals, as well as to undertake what would be a long-term commitment to the physical transformation of the hospital. In fact, Hopkins wanted the biggest safety net it could get when it stepped onto the City Hospitals' ownership tightrope.[93]

More than a decade later, after Schaefer had become Maryland's governor, he would insist that "the hardest bargain... that was ever driven when I was mayor was with Hopkins." At a public ceremony, he waved a finger in mock frustration at Heyssel, who was sitting in the audience, and huffed: "They wanted us to guarantee everything! They wanted a guarantee against lightning striking the building. They wanted a guarantee against floods, and everything. And Heyssel, he kept on saying, 'You know, more, more....'

"So we guaranteed *you*," Schaefer said, pointing his finger again at Heyssel, "that if anything went wrong, if you'd have broken a shoelace, we were going to take the building back. I remember. I know how tough you were."[94]

Talks stalled when agreement could not be reached about the costs that transfer of ownership would entail. At issue was who would cover an estimated $8 million in overdue maintenance costs, and the $50 million to $60 million that would be needed to upgrade or replace the old and often obsolete facilities. Hopkins feared stepping into a bottomless financial pit.[95] Discussions resumed in September 1983 and continued almost weekly until late November, when Benton announced that "for all intents and purposes," the city and Hopkins had concluded the negotiations with an agreement to transfer ownership of City Hospitals to Hopkins.

Talk of an agreement proved premature. Four more months of wrangling were required before Schaefer was able to announce early in March 1984 that the city and Hopkins had, at last, completed the negotiations for the transfer of City Hospitals to Hopkins the following July 1.[96]

Under terms of the agreement, the city promised to pay Hopkins $5.4 million in eight installments over the next four years to cover part of the $8.4 million needed for urgently required maintenance and plant upgrades, and Hopkins said it would loan the remaining $3 million to the city to cover maintenance costs.[97] (Although Hopkins Hospital did guarantee part of the maintenance costs, it met its portion of the upgrade expenses through revenues generated at City Hospitals and never needed to put any of its own money into the facility.[98]) The city and Hopkins also agreed to split 50-50 any profits made from developing land on the hospital grounds for the next 20 years. Finally, the agreement gave Hopkins Hospital the escape hatch Heyssel had wanted: If Hopkins found it could not operate City Hospitals successfully after five years, Hopkins had the right to return it to the city.[99]

Considering the proposal that Hopkins receive all of City Hospitals' assets, assume none of its debts, and be given millions in working capital to fix it "one of the headiest, boldest things ever in my career," Grabill now says he was "just totally shocked that that was an acceptable deal to Benton, Tall, Sondheim, Rosen and the others on that team.

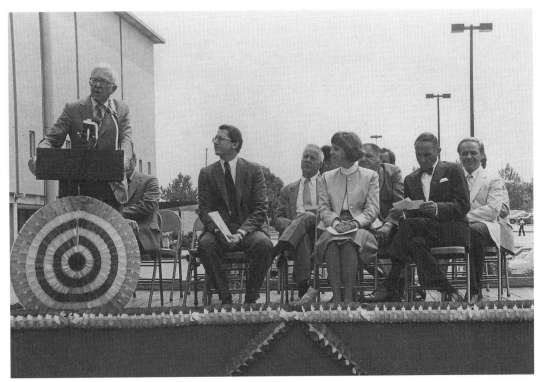

Richard Ross, dean of the Johns Hopkins School of Medicine, speaks at the ceremony marking Hopkins' acquisition of the old City Hospitals on July 2, 1984. On the platform, from the left, are **Ronald R. Peterson,** president of the newly-named Francis Scott Key Medical Center; FSKMC board of trustees chairman **Robert D.H. Harvey; Susan Guarnieri** of the Baltimore City Health Department; City Councilman **Dominic "Mimi" DiPietro;** Edward Halle, vice president for administration of The Johns Hopkins Hospital; and City Councilman **John Schaefer.** (HBBMS)

"It was at that point, as a Hopkins employee, I understood how really badly the city... wanted to get away from the hospital operation, almost at any cost."[100]

A few members of Baltimore's City Council, which had to approve the deal, expressed concerns over it, as did some Southeast Baltimore residents. The community members worried that Hopkins would overbuild on City Hospitals' parklike campus and the green space along its Eastern Avenue boundary would be lost. Councilman Kweisi Mfume (who later would become a member of Congress and then president of the National Association for the Advancement of Colored People) was among those voicing the fear that the poor people being treated at City Hospitals might not receive the same attentive care if Hopkins took over there. Councilman Dominic "Mimi" DiPietro, who represented the First Councilmanic District, in which City Hospitals was located, and who for many years had obtained jobs for his constituents at the facility, had more practical political concerns. "Where is our power?" he asked. If Hopkins took over the hospital, DiPietro wondered aloud, "Are we out of it... ?"[101]

Despite the doubts, on April 16, 1984, the City Council voted 15 to 2 in favor of Bill 180, authorizing the transfer of City Hospitals to Hopkins, with the official takeover set for July 1.[102]

As Colonel Longan had realized 60 years earlier when he changed Bay View Asylum's name to City Hospitals to improve its image, Hopkins faced the problem of taking over an institution that had a grim "traditional image as a municipal hospital for the indigent" and had for years been characterized in the press as "financially plagued" or "financially troubled." ("I knew we were doing better when *The Sun* started to call us 'sprawling,'" quips Philip Zieve.[103])

Hopkins felt a name change was in order, but didn't want to put the Hopkins imprimatur on an institution that still seemed shaky.[104] Ross Jones, a vice president of the university and head of its public affairs office, came up with the idea of calling the facility The Francis Scott Key Medical Center, providing a link to its lengthy history through the name of the Baltimore attorney who had witnessed the British bombardment of Ft. McHenry in 1814 and written "The Star-Spangled Banner" in honor of the fort's survival. The new name "had a community sound to it," Peterson told *The Sun*, and was a "gigantic step away from that negative... image" he was determined to erase.[105]

On a hot and muggy Monday morning, July 2, 1984, Peterson presided over a balloon-bedecked transfer and renaming ceremony featuring a rendering of the national anthem by the Chorus of the Chesapeake and the unveiling of a 12-foot-tall, temporary sign bearing the new name "Francis Scott Key Medical Center" in foot-high letters—and the words "A Johns Hopkins Medical Institution" in much smaller lettering at the bottom, beneath the street address.[106]

"We considered a new name significant," Peterson told the *News American* two days later. Although "the medical folks identify with Baltimore City Hospitals in a positive way, the community generally doesn't," often viewing it as "the welfare hospital." In fact, the hospital provided excellent medical care, he observed, and "so we wanted a positive image—one that has a good association with Baltimore's heritage." He vowed to continue improving the hospital's collection of outstanding debts and to begin planning for "improvement to the physical plant"—a pledge he knew would not be easy to fulfill.[107]

In 1983, in Hopkins' first full fiscal year managing City Hospitals under contract, Peterson and his team wiped out a $6.4 million deficit and put the facility back in the black by $600,000. A region-wide 6 percent reduction in hospital visits that affected all of Maryland's medical facilities in 1983-84—plus a 1984 change in Medicare reimbursement rules for dialysis, cutting payment for that treatment from $1,700 to just $130—pushed City Hospitals back into the red with a $1.6 million loss.[108] By the end of fiscal 1985, the first full year Hopkins owned Francis Scott Key (or FSK, as it became known), the deficit again was pared to just $500,000. The following year, FSK was in the black, recording a $2.6 million "excess of revenues over expenses" (the non-profit accounting term for "profit"), and never again would it dip its bookkeeping pen in red ink.[109]

Peterson "brought to the hospital what it had never had... and that is a knowledge base necessary to run a modern hospital," Zieve says. "And Ron worked harder than any of his predecessors and paid attention to detail in a way that no one ever had before. And the result was that, after the recommendation was made to acquire the hospital, when it was acquired, it was an almost immediate success."

Years later, Schaefer still shook his head in wonder over how Peterson had managed to turn around the hospital that had been a constant headache to him as mayor.

"In the first year, they broke even. And I brought our people in, and my exact words were, 'How the hell can they break even the first year when it cost us a million dollars every year?' And they told me, 'Well, you're not too smart.'

"The second year, he made a profit. And the third year, I knew we'd made a bad deal!"[110]

For Baltimore's oldest continuously operating health care facility, balancing the books for the first time in decades would be just the beginning of an extraordinary transformation.

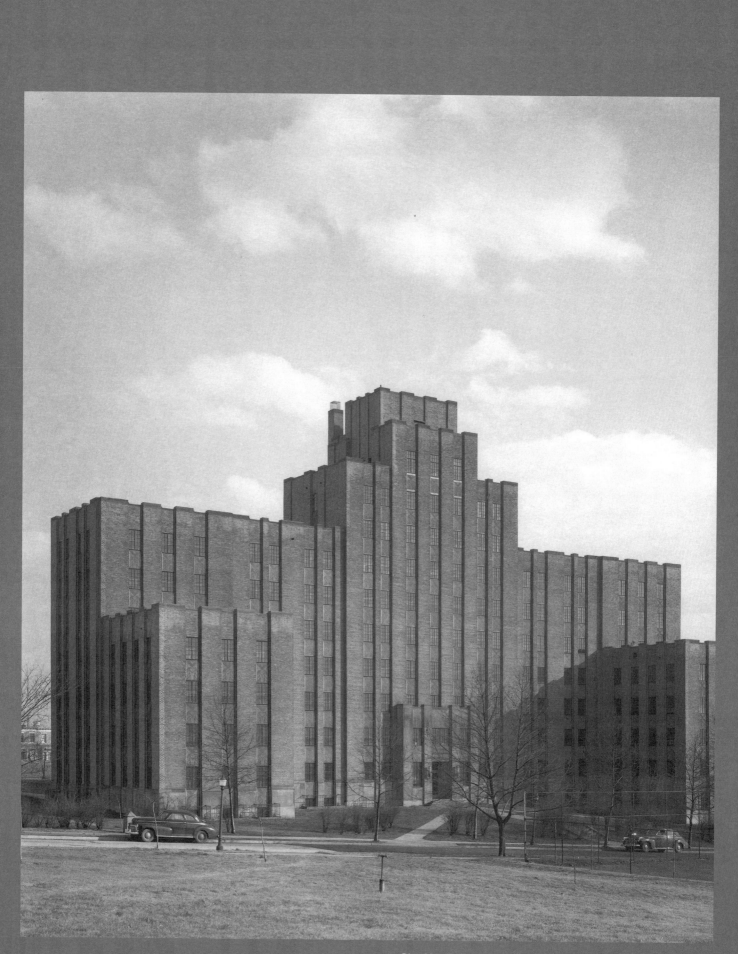

City Hospitals' Nurses' Residence, later the Community Services Center, as it looked in 1947. Its 1989 implosion would become a major community event—and a benchmark of campus revitalization. (HBBMS)

"...A sleeping giant..." 3

I N 1982, THE YEAR JOHNS HOPKINS ASSUMED MANAGEMENT OF Baltimore City Hospitals, the 100 largest cities in the United States had 90 public general hospitals, not counting those owned by universities. These hospitals provided 13.2 percent of inpatient care and 28.9 percent of all hospital outpatient care in those cities.[1]

Twenty years later, only 64 of these municipally supported public general hospitals survived. The last two decades of the 20th century were tumultuous ones for city hospitals, many of which had been in operation for a century or more.[2]

Cities other than Baltimore had been seeking ways to extricate themselves from the hospital business as early as the 1960s. "The growth of health insurance and the advent of Medicare and Medicaid dangled before city hospitals the possibility of paying their own way," Harry F. Dowling observed in his 1982 book, *City Hospitals: The Undercare of the Underprivileged.*

"At the same time, the flight of the upper and middle classes to the suburbs was diminishing the tax base of the cities and of whole metropolitan areas and, by widening the distance between the miseries of the inner city and the comforts of suburbia, was making it harder to extract money from the comfortable to care for the miserable."[3]

Many of these institutions, like Baltimore City Hospitals, were plagued by chronic underfunding. Some were mismanaged by "inefficient, bureaucratic, politically handicapped administrations"; others were alienated from the communities they were supposed to serve, Dowling wrote. Ultimately the control of some city hospitals was handed over to state governments or to private authorities linked to state-owned medical schools; others simply were closed down.[4]

By contrast, the management team that Hopkins sent to Baltimore City Hospitals not only swiftly eliminated its longstanding multimillion-dollar deficits but launched an astounding $100 million transformation of its medical facilities over the next 20 years. In addition to massive renovations of existing facilities, a $15.5 million, 130,000-square-foot geriatrics center was built, followed by a $60 million, 275,000-square-foot acute patient care tower and a

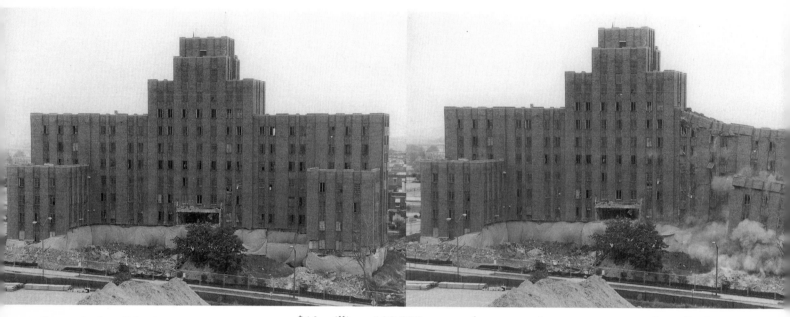

Dramatic demolition by dynamite in August, 1989 of the Community Services Center put an explosive punctuation point on Phase I of the redevelopment project being undertaken by Hopkins on the Francis Scott Key Medical Center campus. (HBBMS)

$13 million, 100,000-square-foot outpatient care center and medical services office building. Outpatient clinic visits went up 80 percent; inpatient admissions soared 86 percent; total surgical procedures increased 87 percent; emergency room visits rose 52 percent. More than 1,800 employees were added to the payroll, and numerous community programs were launched or enhanced.[5]

After nearly two years of managing City Hospitals for Baltimore, Peterson, Grabill and Ward had established a well-honed working relationship. Once Hopkins acquired City Hospitals outright, Peterson became president of the newly christened Francis Scott Key Medical Center (which soon became known simply as FSKMC or FSK), Grabill became vice president for finance and treasurer, and Ward was named vice president for operations and secretary. In November 1984, four months after the acquisition, they were joined by Judy A. Reitz, then 35, as vice president for nursing.[6]

Reitz was born in San Juan, Puerto Rico, where her father, an Army officer, was stationed. She earned her bachelor's and master's degrees in nursing from the University of Maryland School of Nursing. She was a first lieutenant in the U.S. Army Nurse Corps from 1971 to 1973, first at Fort Meade and then at the Walter Reed Army Hospital. Later she was director of Meridian

Healthcare, a regional, long-term care organization, and obtained her doctorate in health finance and management from The Johns Hopkins University School of Hygiene and Public Health while serving as director of nursing practices at Hopkins Hospital.[7]

Under Peterson's leadership, Grabill, Ward and Reitz not only worked well together, but also succeeded in maintaining an unusually strong partnership with the leaders of the Chesapeake Physicians' group, including Zieve, Schmidt, D'Lugoff and Gardner W. Smith. This continued to be a vital collaboration, without which the changes necessary to implement a comprehensive

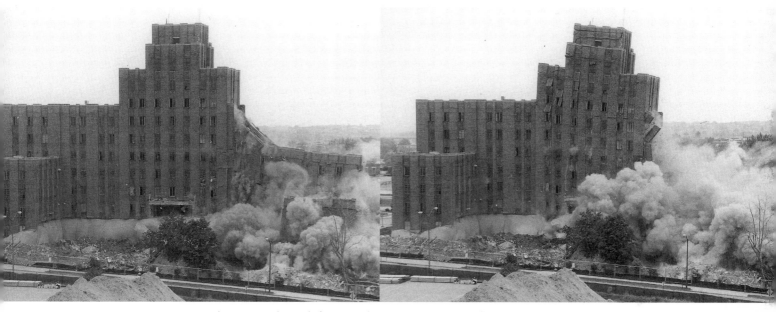

management program to control costs, reduce deficits and increase patient admissions would not have been possible.[8] As Philip Zieve observes, the revitalization was not solely a case of "'these guys from Hopkins came here and they turned it around.'

"They did. But *we* turned it around. They didn't have a prayer without us. We had a prayer without them. They didn't have one idea about clinical program development, for bringing in the next patient. We had already started that by forming the physician group and keeping the hospital alive. The mayor would have closed it years before, probably, except for us. But teaming with Ron and his group, who knew how to get the bills paid and charge properly, and so forth, that's when it really took off."[9]

Despite the hospital's desperate financial situation, Peterson and his vice presidents proceeded carefully and deliberately. "One of the things we focused on, and it turned out in retrospect to be a very important thing to do, was to truly engage the clinical leadership as our partners in planning the redevelopment of the institution, both physically and programmatically," Peterson recalls.[10]

"Rather than go in as a bunch of hospital administrator gunslingers and tell the docs how it was going to be done, we fully engaged them as our partners.

And to this day, I will say to anyone who asks about our success, it was due largely to the fact that we had a wonderful partnership with the people who had been there and understood the nuances of the environment."[11]

Also proving instrumental was an unusually active board of trustees, chaired by Robert D.H. Harvey, chairman of the Maryland National Bank and for 18 years the chairman of The Johns Hopkins University board of trustees. Such civic leaders as attorney William J. McCarthy, developer Francis X. Knott, financial expert W. Wallace Lanahan Jr.—all experienced members of the Hopkins Hospital's board of trustees—agreed, along with Harvey, to

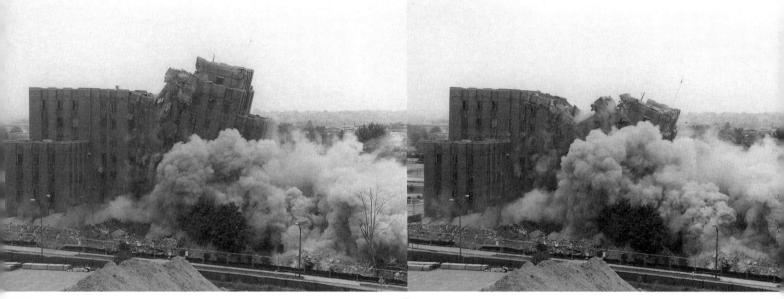

join the Francis Scott Key board. They offered astute advice on such practical matters as establishing good relationships with banks or getting the best billing equipment. The trustees were "able to get the message out about the Hopkins commitment to the activities on this campus," Grabill recalls. "That immediately helped us win the confidence of an awful lot of important players in all the different business transactions that you have to do."[12]

"Basically, what we did was increase the awareness of the downtown business community that there was a Francis Scott Key Medical Center," recalls McCarthy, who would succeed Harvey as chairman of the board. "We got people thinking that in addition to Johns Hopkins, there was another institution way out there in the hinterland that was doing some good work. We saw that it had potential. It was a sleeping giant, you might say."[13]

When FSK later needed to borrow funds to begin the campus's revitalization, the presence on its board of Harvey, McCarthy, Knott and Lanahan, along with others, proved crucial.

"I remember well the first financing we needed," says Francis Knott, another long-time member of The Johns Hopkins University board of trustees. "This was Francis Scott Key Medical Center, this wasn't Johns Hopkins, that was borrowing the money. And Johns Hopkins wasn't on the hook to borrow the money, they weren't the guarantor or anything.

"I remember us meeting with the people from Alex. Brown," Baltimore's venerable and nationally prominent brokerage house. "We had to try to get them to understand that this hospital was on the move, it's headed in the right direction; that's why you should go out and underwrite this issue and help us with the rating agencies."

"The same thing applied to MHHEFA [the Maryland Health and Higher Education Facilities Authority]," Knott explains, "to get them convinced that

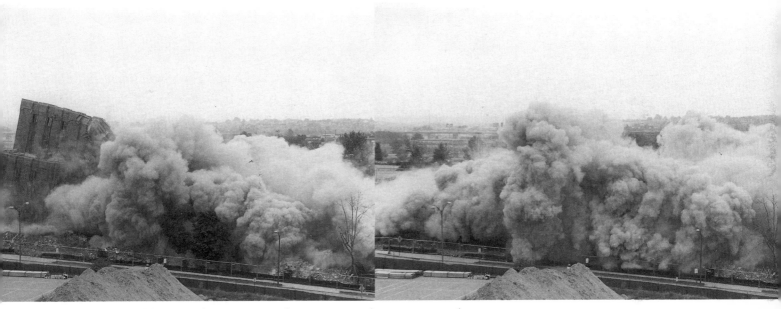

we didn't need 'Daddy' [Hopkins] to sign the guarantee for us to get a loan, that we could do it on our own. And improved financial performance by Francis Scott Key clearly helped that."[14]

The challenge of righting FSK's fiscal ship was proving formidable. Before Hopkins took over, the operating losses of City Hospitals had been more than $6 million annually. In 1984, the last year of city ownership, it provided a record amount of uncompensated care: 11 percent of gross revenue, or nearly $8 million. Such tsunamis of red ink were certain to sink it.[15]

Faced with dramatic pressures both from state regulators and within the health care market itself, the Peterson management team immediately sought to recapture and increase the hospital's patient base; enhance employee productivity (and esprit de corps); reduce costs; and improve such basic automated business systems as the general ledger, accounts payable, billing and personnel.[16]

Recognizing that FSK was not treating enough patients to cover its costs, the Peterson group worked with Chesapeake Physicians' leadership to establish the hospital's first patient-volume targets, as well as a system for monitoring patient care activity.[17] An "Employee Interaction Program" was launched

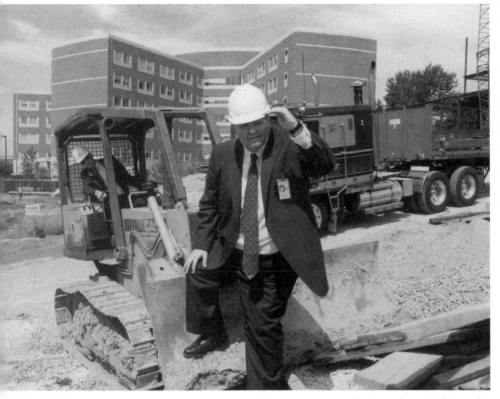

A light look at heavy labor was offered by **Bill Ward**, FSKMC's vice president for operations, manning a bulldozer while **Ken Grabill**, vice president for finance, surveys a construction site during the building boom on the Eastern Avenue campus in the early 1990s. Grabill often spoke of "The Dream" for redevelopment that energized their efforts and the esprit de corps that accompanied it. (HBBMS)

to develop a willingness to serve among hospital workers and encourage them to upgrade their productivity and the quality of their interactions with patients.[18]

When Grabill initially surveyed FSK's financial operations, he found his immediate challenge was to improve the efficiency of the personnel and properly automate the accounting procedures, which still were largely manual due to the inadequacies of the existing computer system.

Even when the process seemed poised to improve, problems occurred. Although Grabill had installed an excellent payroll system, issuance of FSK's first paychecks after Hopkins took over the hospital was inexplicably bollixed by the payroll department staff, whom Grabill characterizes now as "unlucky." The checks were printed, and a die with Grabill's signature was installed in the machine that would sign, stuff and mail the checks. But for some reason the payroll employees "stripped off the pin-feed edges of the 2,000 checks before they had run them through the imprinter," Grabill recalls. "So I literally had to stay up all night and sign 2,000 checks, manually. I got totally cramped up. I didn't have a hand-signature stamp; didn't anticipate that because we had the signature die."[19]

Despite the occasional snafus, Grabill reduced costs significantly by automating the bookkeeping and thereby providing the hospital's managers with their first day-to-day reports on controlling unit costs.

"With timely information, we were able to closely monitor full-time positions and balance them with workloads, reduce overtime, reduce contract nursing services, review all significant supply purchases and plan capital equipment purchases much more effectively," Grabill explained in the hospital's 1985 annual report. Then he oversaw the automation of the patient billing system, immensely improving the hospital's accounts receivable performance.[20]

On the operations front, Ward discovered that the old City Hospitals simply did not have a middle-management group. "It's easy to say, 'start a purchasing function.' It's quite another to find the right people, establish procedures, identify vendors, equipment, telephones and operating systems," Ward observed in the 1985 annual report.[21] He assembled a group of accomplished middle managers and completely overhauled the way the hospital did business. The city's shortsighted, pinch-penny procedures were out.

"Our first emphasis was to change from a philosophy of lowest bid to best value. IV solutions [had been] bought at lowest cost from one supplier, IV tubing from another supplier, and infusion sets [for administering IVs] from still another. The problem was that the tubing was incompatible with the solutions and the infusion sets. We changed to a supplier that could supply all three and thus achieved the best value."[22]

Being united with The Johns Hopkins Hospital also enabled FSK to enter volume-purchasing arrangements with its North Broadway sibling, thereby achieving important economies of scale. Grabill noted in the 1985 annual report, "We are saving $250,000 a year by buying our natural gas for heating directly from a wellhead in Texas, rather than from a local utility."

Judy Reitz took advantage of the affiliation with Hopkins to forge a formal relationship between FSK and the Johns Hopkins School of Nursing. She undertook a "significant restructuring" of the FSK nursing department, integrating the nursing staffs in the acute hospital and the long-term care facility, expanding nurse recruitment to enhance staff leadership, and establishing standards of nursing practice, as well as mechanisms to monitor adherence to them and nursing productivity. She also launched an innovative "career progression system" under which nurses could choose a career track in research, education, administration or clinical practice and advance through different stages on that particular track toward higher levels.[23]

In addition, Reitz landed a $3.5 million grant from the National Institutes of Health to fund the first nursing research program in the country. Under the grant, scientists from the Hopkins School of Medicine worked with nurse investigators at FSK to study the impact of disease on aging, exploring such issues as pain management and factors that influence diet and weight control in seniors.[24]

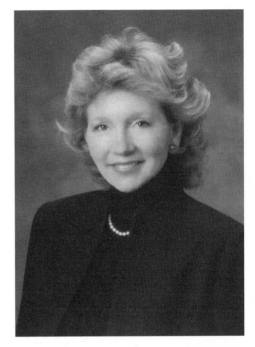

Judy Reitz joined the Peterson management team at **FSKMC** in November 1984 as vice president for nursing. By 1993, she had become executive vice president and chief operating officer for **FSKMC** and later would return to Hopkins Hospital as senior vice president for operations when Ronald Peterson became its president. (Above, Johns Hopkins Medicine Office of Corporate Communications [JHMOCC]; below left, HBBMS)

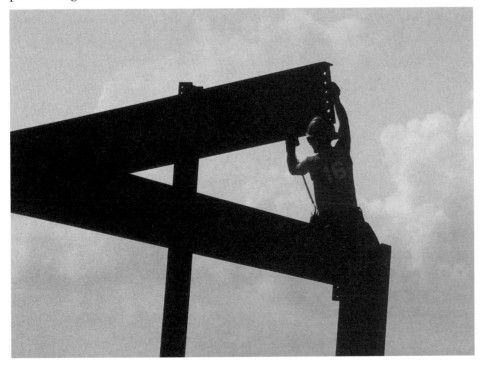

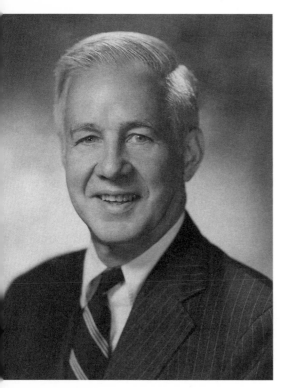

Long-time trustees of The Johns Hopkins Hospital, (left to right) banker **Robert D.H. Harvey,** attorney **William McCarthy,** real estate developer **Francis X. Knott** and financier **Wallace Lanahan,** agreed in 1984 to assume additional duties on the Francis Scott Key Medical Center board of trustees. Harvey as chairman, McCarthy as vice chairman, Knott as head of the building committee and Lanahan succeeded in persuading Baltimore's business community that FSKMC had a promising future and merited financial support. Harvey remains on the Hopkins Bayview board today; McCarthy is now chairman, and Knott still leads the building committee. (Above and opposite, The Johns Hopkins University Board of Trustees; left, Mike Ciesielski)

In initiating their reorganization of FSK, Peterson and his associates were alert to the fact that they were setting out to effect a major culture change and alter the ingrained habits of a workforce that had been made up of municipal employees for two centuries. They knew they had some time-servers on their staff, but they also knew they had a core of dedicated employees who were proud of where they worked and what they did. A scalpel, not a meat-axe, was the right surgical tool for the winnowing operation.

"Although we were not shy about jettisoning some of the poor performers, we did not go in there with the attitude that we would cause the city employees to be forced out en masse," Peterson says. "We only caused changes to occur selectively, rather than displace the whole bloody crew. Because of that, we were able to get the respect of the people who were there. Whenever any larger, more sophisticated organization is taking over another, you have to be sensitive to these things. And I think that really worked to our benefit."[25]

The Peterson team did its best to counter what they privately labeled "the school bus syndrome" among the hospital's veteran former city employees. "There was this sense that one day, a whole bunch of school buses were going to show up, and a bunch of Hopkins folks were going to get off, and the folks from [the old] City [Hospitals] were going to get on—and they'd never be seen again," Ward recalls. "We literally fought that for years."[26]

Ward began the practice of "VP Coffees," an opportunity scheduled four times a year for employees to meet with one of the hospital's vice presidents at any time during a 24-hour period, with the VPs trading shifts to cover an entire day. "So any worker in any shift got a VP for a day. They could go to the session and ask anything they wanted, get information on what Ken used to call 'The Dream,' which was the redevelopment [planning]," Ward

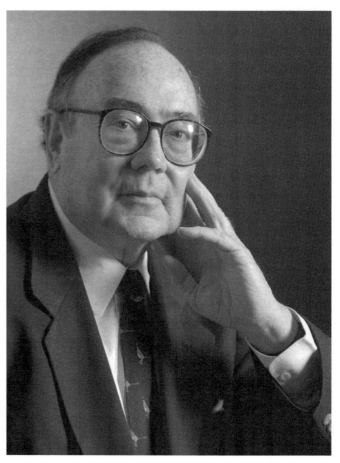

says. He adds, with a sigh, "You always got the question: 'How are you going to do the layoff?' We never had one."[27]

A good example of how carefully FSK's leadership handled labor relations was the way they decided to close the hospital's venerable but terribly outdated and costly laundry. The two-floor facility would have required immense capital investment to replace its aging equipment and undertake major building renovations. Every effort was made to avoid laying off any of its 60 to 70 employees, many of whom had been there for decades.

"We knew we were going to close it, but we didn't close it right away," Ward explains. Under a provision of the agreement giving Hopkins control of the hospital, employees who wanted to stay on the city payroll were given a limited time in which to leave their jobs at FSK and take another city job with no loss in seniority. "And so every time that happened, we hired a temp," Ward says. "We hired temps in dietary; we hired temps for the grounds departments; we hired temps in housekeeping and so on—any place we thought a laundry worker could be trained to take that position."

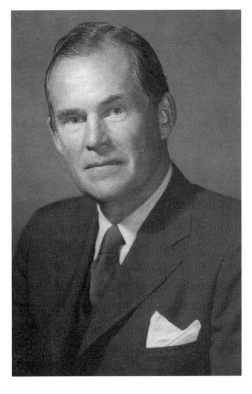

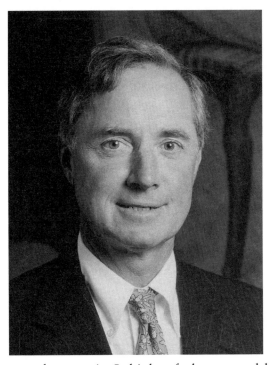

Once there were enough of these open positions to which laundry employees could be transferred, Ward and others told the laundry workers that their shop was closing, but they all would be retrained and would continue as FSK employees. Ward remembers that a leader of the employees' union "turned to me and said, 'We've never had an employer do this. They don't look out for workers.' And that was the genesis, I think, of phenomenal labor relations there. Because the workers saw that we recognized their value, that they weren't just supplies or pieces of equipment, but real people who looked out for people."[28]

FSK began to see its patient volume rise steadily, thanks in no small part to the leadership's collaboration with Chesapeake Physicians. As Maryland's largest private, multipractice specialty medical group (with 150 full-time and 60 part-time physicians), CPPA already was skilled at community outreach.[29] Ambulatory (outpatient) surgeries nearly doubled, from 75 in 1984 to almost 150 in 1985; and all other surgical procedures increased as well, growing from 4,759 in 1985 to 5,016 in 1987.[30] Admissions to the acute care hospital also rose steadily, growing by 300 in 1985 to a total of 10,964.

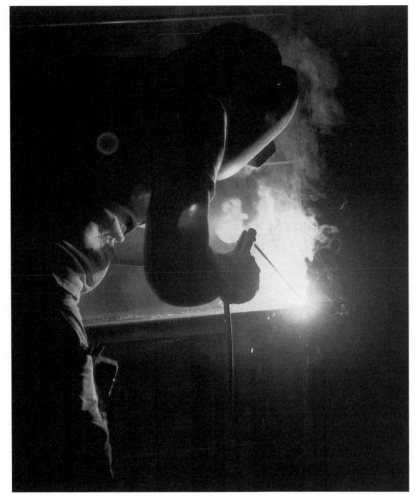

Targeted for closure in a 1982 consultant's report, the Eastern Avenue hospital that became Hopkins Bayview instead experienced a construction spree that has made it among the most modern medical facilities in the region. (HBBMS)

By 1989, admissions had risen by almost 2,000, reaching 12,931 by the end of that fiscal year.[31]

Not long before Hopkins took over management of City Hospitals in 1982, the state of Maryland had hired the management consulting firm of Booz, Allen & Hamilton to study hospital capacity in Maryland. The resulting report quickly was dubbed "The Hit List" in the medical community, since it named the institutions that Booz, Allen & Hamilton deemed expendable—and City Hospitals was one. But one year after Hopkins took over complete control of the institution, Peterson was proud to report in the new institutional magazine, *Keynotes,* that the "most significant" development in the first year of Hopkins' ownership was that FSK no longer was "targeted for closure" in the latest Booz, Allen & Hamilton assessment of Maryland's hospitals.[32]

Even before formulating a master plan for redevelopment of the FSK campus, Peterson promptly sought to upgrade the institution's image by making "cosmetic improvements" in the major public areas and patient care facilities. Even these modest efforts were greeted with excitement. "It was a great boon to the campus," recalls John Burton, the long-time chief of geriatrics. "Suddenly we had something happening! We saw a dump truck for the first time in 30 years!"[33]

The master planning process got under way in June 1985, the same month in which the National Institute on Drug Abuse, pleased with the improvements on the campus apparent since Hopkins' takeover, followed through on its anticipated expansion there and opened its newly renovated Addiction Research Center.[34]

To assist in the master planning, Peterson put together an architectural, engineering and financing team by hiring RTKL, a Baltimore-based architectural firm with well-demonstrated health care expertise, as well as engineering savvy; the New York-based engineering firm of Joseph R. Loring and Associates, and representatives of the Ernst and Whinney accounting and financial services company (precursor of today's firm of Ernst and Young).[35]

Peterson also formed the Medical Center Clinical Program Planning Committee that included Zieve, Schmidt, Smith, D'Lugoff and William R. Furman, as well as Reitz and Ward. Their goal was major revitalization of the hospital's physical plant, and they explored every option, from tearing down all the buildings and starting over to renovating and retrofitting the existing structures.[36] Whatever was done had to improve not only the look of the facilities but their efficiency.

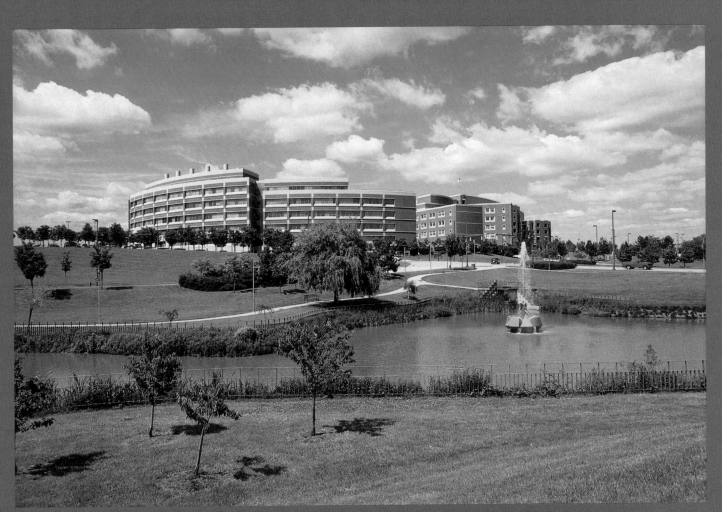

Green space preservation was a vital concern of the Southeast Baltimore community when Johns Hopkins acquired the old City Hospitals. The hospital worked closely with the community to design this 10-acre "passive urban park" with a pond, walking and jogging paths and new landscaping on the sloping greensward that stretches down the hill to Eastern Avenue in front of the campus. (HBBMS)

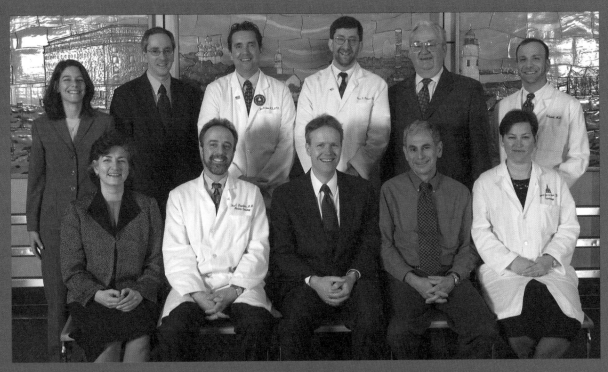

Among the leaders of the Hopkins Bayview Department of Medicine are (seated, left to right) **Linda P. Fried,** chief, geriatric medicine and gerontology; **Roy S. Ziegelstein,** executive vice chairman, medicine; **David Hellmann,** chair, medicine, and physician-in-chief; **Gary Briefel,** chief, renal medicine; **Suzanne Jan de Beur,** chief, endocrinology, (standing, left to right), **Melissa Feld,** administrator for medicine; **Antony Rosen,** chief of rheumatology; **John Stone,** deputy director of clinical research; **Bruce Bochner,** chief of allergy and clinical immunology; **Donald Jasinski,** chief of chemical dependency; **Steven Kravet,** deputy director for clinical activities and director of the Collaborative Inpatient Medical Service. (Kevin Weber)

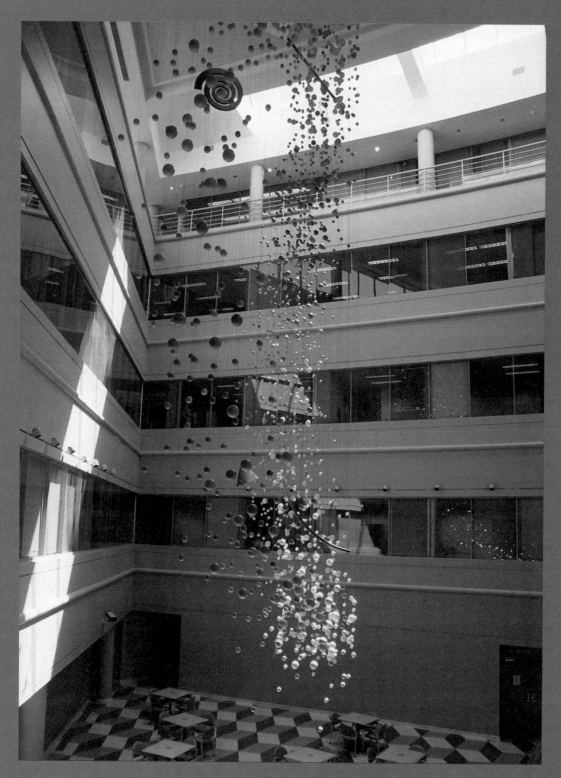

"The Big Sneeze" is the unofficial title bestowed by employees on this eclectic sculpture in the spacious five-story atrium of the Asthma & Allergy Center of the Johns Hopkins School of Medicine on the Hopkins Bayview campus. Created by Oregon artist Larry Kirkland, the colorful assemblage of painted maple, steel and aluminum actually is entitled *Aspirato*, the Latin word for "I breathe." Kirkland says it was inspired by his personal physician, who has asthma. Right, **Philip Zieve** confers with young physicians. (HBBMS)

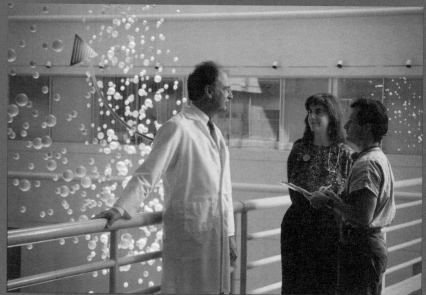

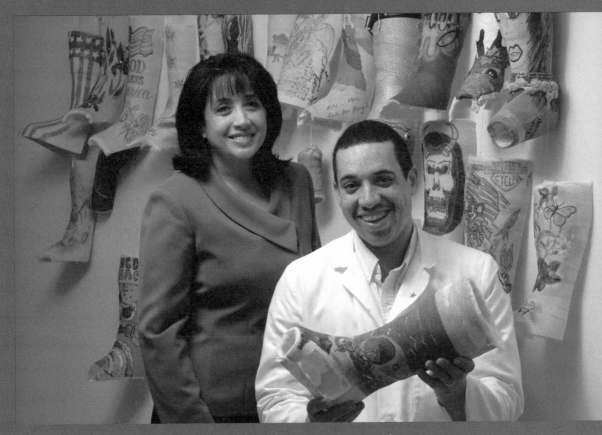

Colorful casts decorated by orthopedic patients at Hopkins Bayview form a creative display in the office of orthotist Michael Keene, right, shown here with Hayat Nesheiwat, nurse manager. Keene and his colleague Rob Rawson evaluate, fit and measure patients for assistive and support devices including casts. Keene says that although assembling casts is "fun and interesting," the most satisfying moments in his work come when they are removed "and the patient says 'I'm healed.'" (Mike Ciesielski)

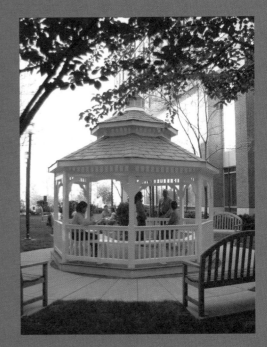

A quiet place to relax and converse is the gazebo in Hopkins Bayview's Gaston Courtyard. The gazebo is a memorial to James Wenz, a brilliant orthopedic surgeon, and his wife, Lidia Wenz, a child psychiatrist, who were killed in an auto accident in January 2004. (Mike Ciesielski)

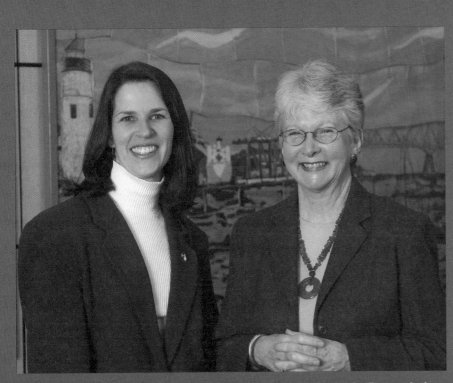

Maureen M. Gilmore, left, chair, neonatology, and **Dorothy L. Rosenthal,** chair, pathology. (Kevin Weber)

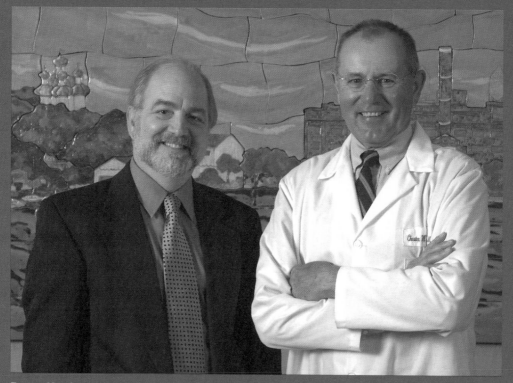

Peter Kaplan, left, chair, neurology, and **Chester Schmidt,** chair, psychiatry. (Kevin Weber)

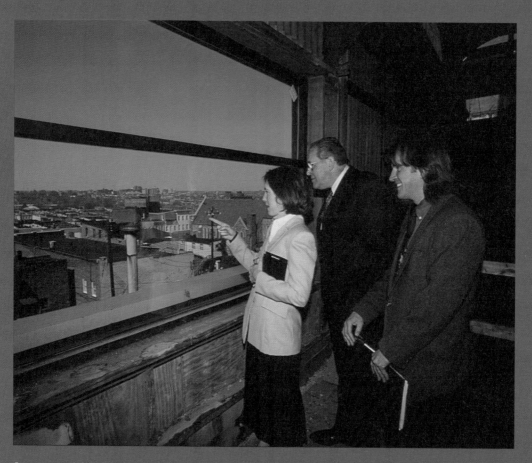

A room with a view enables Hopkins Bayview president Greg Schaffer, who also is chairman of the Southeast Community Development Corporation (SCDC), to see "areas of opportunity" for enhancing Highlandtown as SCDC president CEO Michele Decker and John Lundquist point them out. Decker says Hopkins Bayview "puts money on the table and volunteers the time and wisdom of its leadership" as well as "offers a market for us in its employees, who are potential homeowners and customers" in the area. (HBBMS)

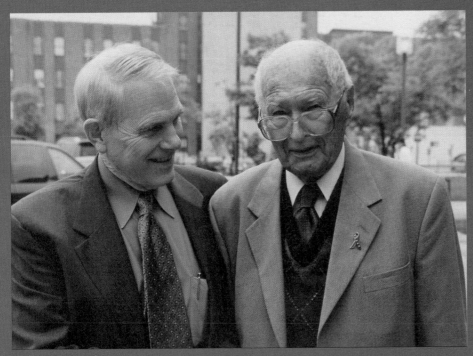

Generations of gerontologists: **John Burton,** left, with 89-year-old **Edmund Beacham** at the 2003 renaming of the Hopkins Bayview geriatrics building as the John R. Burton Pavilion, recognizing Burton's decades of leadership of the programs that Beacham helped to found. (HBBMS)

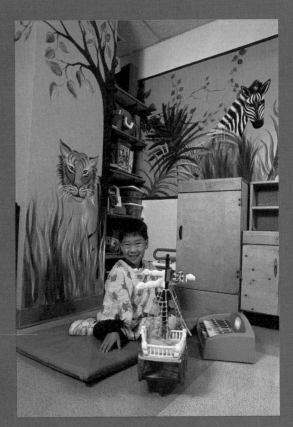

Wild things decorate the playroom in the Hopkins Bayview Department of Pediatrics inpatient center. (HBBMS)

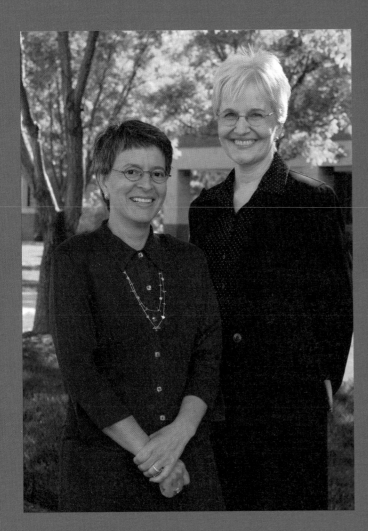

Maria Koszalka, Ed. D., vice president, patient care services, and **Anita M. Lanford, vice president,** continuing care, are instrumental in maintaining Hopkins Bayview's tradition of compassionate care. (Mike Ciesielksi)

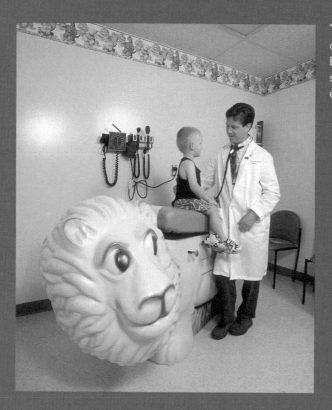

The friendly atmosphere of a neighborhood pediatric office prevails in the Children's Medical Practice at Hopkins Bayview under **Michael Crocetti,** chief of pediatrics, shown here with a patient perched atop a grinning lion examination table. (HBBMS)

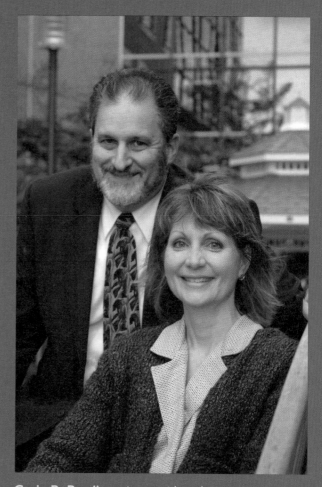

Craig R. Brodian, vice president, human resources, and **Michele T. Lagana,** vice president, administration, are among Hopkins Bayview's new generation of leaders. (Mike Ciesielski)

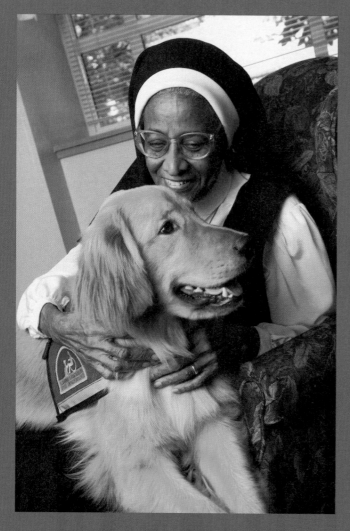

Therapeutic pooch: Selby, a specially trained golden retriever, is an enormously popular member of Hopkins Bayview's ElderPlus program staff. He even has his own staff ID card. His gentle, loving nature helps promote the physical and mental health of ElderPlus patients such as **Sister Corde Marie Gonzalez.** A gift to ElderPlus from Canine Companions for Independence, a nonprofit group, Selby can turn lights on and off, open and close doors, and help patients get out of chairs. Selby's most important role, says physical therapy assistant Anne Fraim, is as the program's "best motivator. He gets participants moving and interacting with one another." (HBBMS)

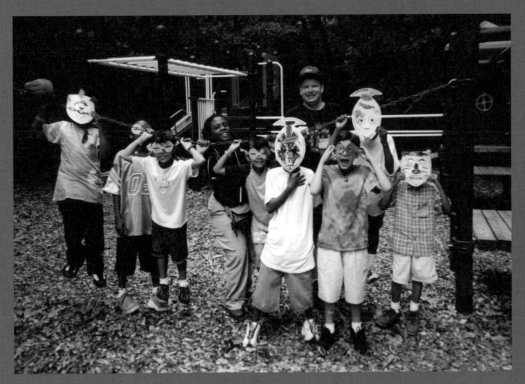

Happy campers at Camp Superkids, a week-long overnight camp for children with asthma, display masks they created during arts and crafts time. The camp is underwritten by Hopkins Bayview and the American Lung Association of Maryland and staffed by nurses, respiratory therapists, physician assistants, counselors and non-medical personnel. (HBBMS)

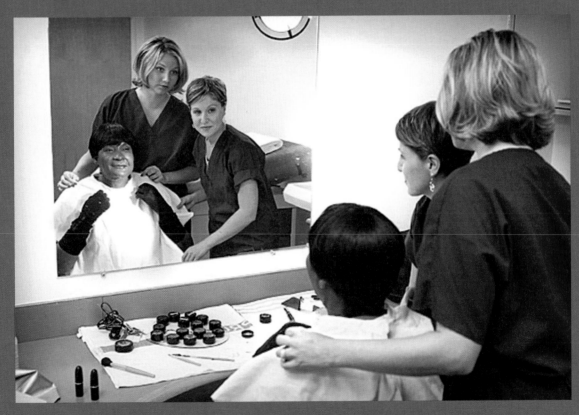

Corrective cosmetics came to Hopkins Bayview in 2002, when it became the first hospital on the East Coast to offer such care as part of the Center for Burn Reconstruction's comprehensive image and behavior enhancement program for burn survivors. Here, physical therapist **Debra Stillman** (on the right in mirror) and occupational therapist **Michelle Ober** help a patient learn how to apply special cosmetics developed in Hollywood to even out discoloration caused by scars and redness resulting from skin grafts. (HBBMS)

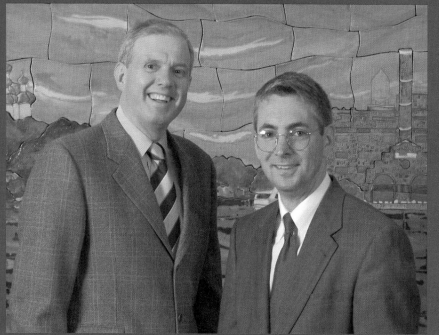

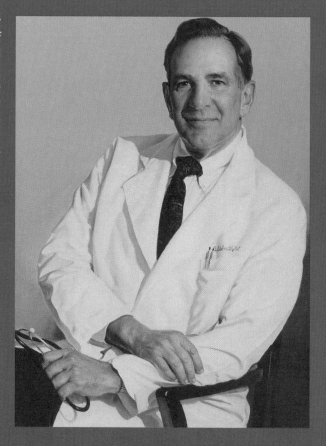

Alessandro Olivi, chairman of neurosurgery, and Mark D. Duncan, interim chairman of surgery. (Kevin Weber)

Gardner W. Smith was Surgeon-in-Chief at the Baltimore City Hospitals from July 1970 to March 1979. He then served as Chairman of the Section of Surgical Sciences at the Johns Hopkins Bayview Medical Center from June 1985 to June 1996. From March 1979 to June 1985, Smith was Deputy Director of the Department of Surgery at Johns Hopkins Hospital. His leadership was instrumental in the success of the transition from city ownership of the hospital to its affiliation with Johns Hopkins. He now is an emeritus professor of surgery in the Hopkins School of Medicine, and a lectureship in surgery is named in his honor. (Painting by Peter Egeli, 1996)

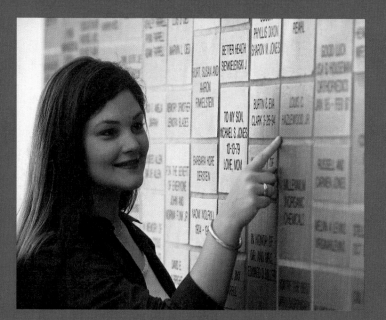

The Wall of Caring in the Francis Scott Key Pavilion is made of bricks bearing the names of grateful community members and organizations that have donated funds to Hopkins Bayview. (HBBMS)

Previously, "new departments and services went where there was empty space, not where they should have been located for efficient operation," Ward observed at the time. Cardiology, for instance, was located on three different floors in three different buildings, two of which were on opposite sides of the sprawling, 263,000-square-foot acute care complex: the A Building, opened in 1935 and added to in 1949 and 1968, the AA ("Acute Addition") Building, opened in 1965, and the B-South Building, erected in 1908.[37]

In *Keynotes,* Ward stressed that employees across the campus would be involved in the master planning. "By no means will this be an autocratic procedure. It will sort out a wealth of information from inside and outside the institution. I'm sure we'll see a diverse number of creative solutions incorporated into final plans. These will bring us significant benefits.

"Redevelopment can make us more efficient in our operations, which certainly translates into lower costs," Ward said. "This whole process can help us to improve our public image, make us more cost-competitive and attract more patients—and that translates into lower costs, too."[38]

Improving FSK's public image and combating its lingering reputation as the "welfare hospital," compounded now by the seeming remoteness of its Hopkins owners, required cultivating the residents of the hospital's own neighborhood.

To bolster community outreach, FSK's Community Advisory Board, a committee of local leaders that had been disbanded when the city relinquished ownership of the hospital, was re-established. Peterson often met directly with this board to develop personal relationships, and he went into the community, attending neighborhood meetings and giving speeches, to make himself accessible to the area's residents in ways his predecessors had not done.[39] He created the new position of director of community relations and promoted Gayle Johnson Adams, an experienced social worker who had joined the hospital's staff in 1974, to fill it. Adams had for many years been the face of City Hospitals at neighborhood association meetings. Her elevation demonstrated that Peterson recognized the importance of her work, and it impressed the community groups with which she was familiar.

"I'm not trying to blow my own horn, but it helped him [Peterson] to have somebody in place whom the community already trusted," says Adams, a native Baltimorean. "They knew they were going to get a straight story from me, and for me to be able to say 'You can deal with Ron, you can trust what he's telling you' was helpful for the new administration coming in from Hopkins. For the community to see that I was still here, that I actually was promoted, reporting directly to the president, said to them that the community is important to this guy."[40]

In re-establishing the community advisory board, Adams recalls, she tried to recruit members who were leaders in more than one sector of the community so she "could have 15 people in the room but reach 30 or 40

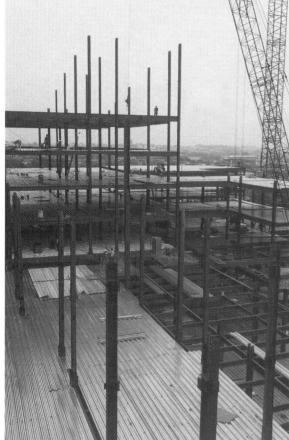

A forest of girders sprouted on Eastern Avenue during the late 1980s and 1990s. (HBBMS)

groups, because they were people who owned a business and belonged to a service club or a church and [also] were active in their community association."[41]

Originally a community relations department of one, Adams oversaw the steady expansion of her activities and the growth of her staff. As planning for the revitalization of the campus began in 1985, she participated closely in the process and kept the neighborhood organizations surrounding the hospital fully informed of what was being considered. Doing so meant going to the groups' night or weekend meetings, or inviting leaders of the community to the hospital for regular updates.

"The community just east of the hospital didn't have a community organization back then," Adams recalls, "so we would have meetings here at the hospital and invite them in. Either Ron or Bill Ward would participate, talk to them about what our plans were, what we wanted to do, get their feedback, find out what the problems were going to be with the plans," such as traffic disruptions due to the demolition of old buildings and the erection of new ones.[42]

FSK staff became even more involved in community activities and sought to use its influence to help area residents address concerns that did not directly affect health care, such as police, fire protection, and other "crime, grime and education" matters that were their daily priorities. "Our role has always been, if it's the community's problem, it's ours, too," says Adams. "Politically, if we want community support when we have an issue, when we need the community's help in advocating for resources or legislation or whatever, we need to be there when they have [issues]. We can't just come and take from the community, we have to give back to it."[43]

Several new programs were enhanced or created, including the Southeast Emergency Needs Network, which maintained an emergency food closet to provide groceries for the needy; an intermediate care unit, a GI Pain Center and a Center for Chemical Dependence with a full range of substance abuse services.[44]

Meetings were held with the Bayview Civic Association, the 15th Street Improvement Association and other groups representing the communities surrounding the hospital's campus. The area's residents wanted to be sure that the green space in front of the hospital would be preserved. Both the medical center and the Dome Corporation, a for-profit, business development entity created in 1984 by The Johns Hopkins Hospital and University, worked closely with FSK's neighbors to develop the design for a 10-acre "passive urban park" with a pond, walking and jogging paths, and new landscaping on the sloping greensward that stretched down the hill to Eastern Avenue in front of the Mason F. Lord Building. Perry Sfikas, then president of the Bayview Civic Association (and later a Maryland state senator representing Southeast Baltimore), voiced his group's satisfaction with the outcome. "I have to say we were not only impressed with the kind of park the hospital proposed, which is beautiful, but the way they worked with us and fulfilled their obligation. They're good neighbors," he told an FSK publication, *Community News*.[45]

"I think [community] people started to believe more" in Hopkins' management once the green space was preserved and embellished as a park, Adams says.

Banking on its position as the only hospital in the Southeast Baltimore community, FSK's new leaders hoped these initiatives would help enhance its image in the neighborhood, attract more patients, and thus enable it to ride out its financial storms and survive.[46] But neighbors' complete comfort with the new owner of the hospital still was a long way off.[47]

Overall, the master planning process produced ambitious goals. These included demolishing the 120-year-old Lord Building and the 54-year-old, nine-story Community Service Building, originally a nurses' residence; construction of a new comprehensive geriatrics facility; redeveloping the acute care hospital and long-term care facility; erecting an ambulatory care center and medical office building; and developing a comprehensive biomedical technology research campus that could include a small hotel and conference center.[48]

Some of those buildings would never go up; one, the Mason F. Lord Building, would not come down—literally. It was a typical example of mid-19th century institutional architecture, built to last, with walls that in some places were 18 inches thick. Demolition costs would be astronomical. (During a February 1953 renovation, a construction worker had found a pair of boots buried in a portion of a wall there. Inside one of the boots was a note that read "buried in October 1868" and bearing the signature "Cassell." The first name was illegible, but research showed that a man named Cassell was one of the founders of the local bricklayers' union in 1866. The road leading from Eastern Avenue to the building then was named Cassell Drive in his honor.[49])

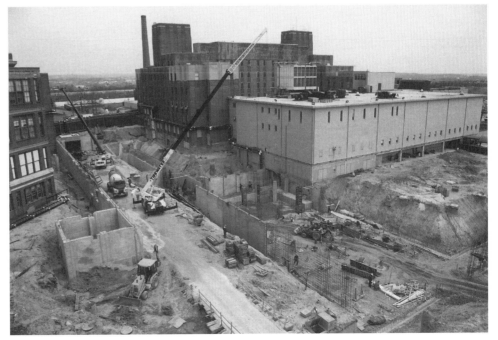

Dig we must. Construction crews in 1991 excavate a foundation for what would become the Francis Scott Key Pavilion of the Johns Hopkins Bayview Medical Center. **(HBBMS)**

The original plan called for the Lord Building's demolition by 1987, but its date with the wrecker's ball kept being postponed. The Dome Corporation anticipated developing a $500 million biomedical research park on the west side of the FSK campus, where the Lord Building stood. That goal made construction of a long-term care facility (the geriatrics center) a priority, to establish a new home for patients still housed in the Lord Building. Once

Bulldozers and construction cranes became common sights on the Francis Scott Key Medical Center campus. The new and old are captured in this 1988 photo of the Johns Hopkins School of Medicine's Asthma & Allergy Center under construction, with the 1931 Community Services Center, slated for implosion, in the distance. (HBBMS)

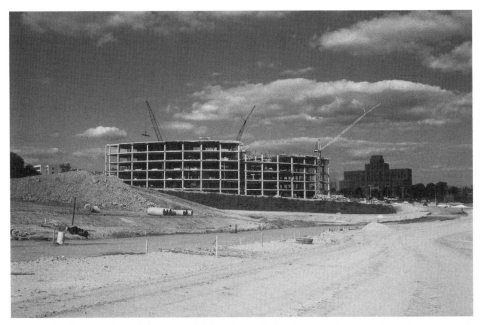

emptied, the Lord Building could be demolished to make way for the research park. The redevelopment financial planners seemed puzzled. "The folks who were looking at the bond underwriting were saying 'Build the cash cow, the acute [care] building first, and then you can fund this other stuff'," Ward recalls. "We really did the opposite. But part of it was driven by the development plan, and so that led to Phase I being the geriatrics center."[50]

Ultimately, the Dome Corporation was unable to develop the biomedical research park project as rapidly as it had anticipated, and the now-emptying Lord Building proved to be an excellent and extremely cost-efficient source of "incubator" space for developing companies. So instead of demolishing the 364,000-square-foot, seven-million-brick behemoth, it was decided that as other new structures went up and the services once housed in the Lord Building moved into them, a complete renovation would be launched inside the old warhorse. In time it became the home of some of the finest modern laboratories and other facilities for the Johns Hopkins School of Medicine.[51]

"We emptied the Mason Lord Building out and, guess what, it's still there—and it will be there after the roaches and ivy and everything else are gone from the planet," Ward says with a chuckle.

In addition to construction of the new geriatrics care facility, Phase I of the master plan included a desperately needed new central utilities plant (CUP), demolition of the Community Services Center, and a limited renovation of the existing medical facilities. The initial estimate for the costs of Phase I was $36 million. Phase II would include construction of a new inpatient tower, demolition of the B-South Building, erected in 1908, and major renovations and retrofitting of the acute hospital, last updated 20 years earlier. The estimated cost of this phase was $57.2 million.[52]

Although most of the planning was completed by the end of 1986, the need to pay for its proposals was another significant hurdle. An impressive demonstration of FSK's ability to remain consistently in the black was the key to financing the multimillion-dollar debt that would have to be undertaken to fund the construction projects.[53]

After Maryland's Health Services Cost Review Commission had been persuaded in late 1982 to raise the hospital's rates significantly, it kept a close eye on its operations. Over the next three years, the commission's methodology for comparing FSK's finances with those of its urban peer group changed, and in October 1985, the HSCRC decided FSK was not "as efficient" in curbing patient care costs as its urban hospital peers, Grabill recalls. Its rates were deemed to be 9.4 percent higher than the average charges of similar institutions. After negotiations, the commission reached a settlement with FSK in November that required the hospital to lower its "high-cost" rates by 4.5 percent to 5 percent.

"It was a challenge," Grabill says. "It was a hard reality test at the time, make no mistake about that."

Most fixed costs of operating any hospital—electricity, heat, management—can remain much the same no matter how much patient volume is generated, Grabill explains. Only variable costs, such as supplies and nursing hours, can be adjusted. The challenge was to constrain those costs and increase patient volume as much as possible.

"We did some of both," Grabill says, "but we especially did an excellent job of bringing on volume, raising productivity in the workforce."[54]

The cost-cutting and business efficiency procedures implemented by the Peterson team combined with the energetic patient outreach activities of Chesapeake Physicians paid off impressively. Patient admissions grew some 8 percent or 9 percent annually, or about 1,000 more each year than they had in the last days of city-run administration. And the collection rate soared. "Every percentage point on the collection rate here is equal to $800,000 on our bottom line," Peterson noted in 1987. Collections rose from about 79 percent to 85 percent during the first two full years of Peterson's presidency, making a considerable impact on the ledger. By the summer of 1987, FSK was projecting a $5 million profit.[55]

Impressed and pleased as Robert Heyssel was with the Peterson team's performance at FSK, he continued to be concerned about the increasing competitiveness in the health care industry. Freestanding hospitals appeared to face a perilous future. Individual consumers, their employers and their insurers were complaining about rising health care costs and demanding that they be curbed. One way to do that was to create shared programs in purchasing, contract management, clinical planning and malpractice insurance to achieve economies of scale. A unified system also would provide broader access to capital markets, something that both FSK and The Johns Hopkins Hospital would need to launch redevelopment projects.[56]

In the spring of 1986, Heyssel announced the formation of the Johns Hopkins Health System (JHHS), which comprised The Johns Hopkins Hospital, the Francis Scott Key Medical Center, and three other health care providers then associated with Hopkins. These were the North Charles General Hospital in Charles Village in Baltimore, which became affiliated with Hopkins in November 1985; the Wyman Park Health System, located in a former U.S. Public Health Service hospital beside Hopkins' Homewood campus, which became affiliated with Hopkins in March 1986; and the Johns Hopkins Health Plan, a health maintenance organization (HMO) created by Hopkins in 1985. With its four hospitals and its HMO's 15 health plan sites, the new JHHS immediately became one of the largest nonprofit health care providers in the country.[57]

The composition of JHHS would change over the years. North Charles General Hospital eventually would be closed, and other groups and hospitals, such as Howard County General Hospital, would be added, but FSK would remain a central contributor to the system's vitality and growth.

Gradual change in the self-image of FSK's former city employees was reflected in their decision in May 1986 to end their affiliation with the labor union that had represented them, the Classified Municipal Employees Association (CMEA). More than 500 of FSK's 2,100 employees had been CMEA members since the late 1950s. They were white-collar workers in technical, clerical and secretarial positions, as well as such professionals as therapists, social workers, dietitians and physician's assistants. Their union had bargained for them with Baltimore city for nearly 30 years.[58]

Early in 1986, about 30 percent of the CMEA-represented employees who worked in FSK's acute care hospital and long-term care facility filed a petition with the National Labor Relations Board (NLRB) seeking to end their association with the union. They said they preferred to deal directly with Peterson's management team, rather than through an intermediary.[59]

An initial vote on April 29 was inconclusive. The NLRB ballot offered three choices: no union; retention of CMEA representation; and membership in two other intervening unions, the Service Employees International Union (SEIU) and the United Food and Commercial Workers (UFCW), both affiliates of the AFL-CIO. None of the ballot alternatives received a majority, so a second vote was held on May 29, with the ballot limited to two choices: retention of CMEA representation and "no union." By a vote of 218 to 211, the CMEA lost. It was a gratifying outcome for Peterson's team despite the razor-thin margin of victory.

"We view the decertification petition by our employees and the subsequent outcome of the NLRB election as a vote of confidence in the hospital management team," Peterson said after the balloting. "Their decision is to deal directly with the management team, rather than to be represented by a third party. We are very pleased with their decision."[60]

In May 1987, the 390 registered nurses who constituted FSK's largest group of professional employees followed suit, voting 163-106 to decertify the Maryland Nurses Association (MNA) as their collective bargaining representative, ending a 21-year association.

Ward was so proud of the employees' vote to drop their unions—and what that said about FSK management's efforts to improve labor relations—that he kept copies of the decertification notices framed in his office at home.[61]

Along with improving employee morale, Peterson recognized the importance of cultivating political connections on behalf of the medical center. He'd actually received a valuable lesson in the fine art of constituent service years earlier when, as a young administrative resident at Hopkins Hospital in 1973, he had tagged along with vice president for administration Robert Wilson to an event held at City Hospitals as part of its bicentennial celebration. It was his first trip to the campus he would later rejuvenate, and a memorably instructive one.

After a presentation at the hospital's Carroll Auditorium, Wilson and Peterson proceeded to a reception at the cafeteria, where Peterson saw a long line already assembled. "I assumed it was a line for the food, but what it turned out to be was a line of people waiting to see [city councilman Dominic] Mimi DiPietro," Peterson recalls. "Well, it was almost like something out of 'The Godfather,' because some people would kiss his ring—I mean, he was 'The Mayor of Highlandtown'! And that stuck with me. And when I went over there in '82, every once in a while, Mimi DiPietro would call me when he wanted a job for somebody. It was the old school of politics."[62]

Once he became president of FSK, Peterson made certain that the politicians who represented the hospital's community received full credit for whatever help they provided to the institution. He regularly scheduled award presentations to honor local legislators and others who sought government grants and similar sources of funding for FSK programs. In 1986 alone, he presented commemorative plaques to Maryland State Senators Joseph Bonvegna and Thomas Bromwell, Delegates American Joe Miedusiewski and Charles (Bucky) Muth, and leaders of the International Association of Fire Fighters and the Maryland/D.C. Professional Fire Fighters Association for their help in landing a $250,000 state grant to expand and renovate the Baltimore Regional Burn Center at FSK. At every groundbreaking or ribbon-cutting ceremony at the medical center, Peterson personally recognized the presence of politicos in the audience.[63]

The expanded community outreach and comprehensive master planning reflected one facet of the vitality of the Francis Scott Key campus since the

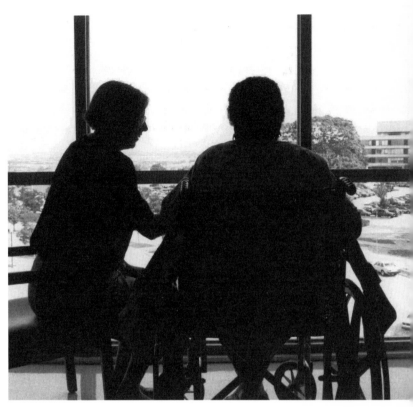

Panoramic views of Baltimore are provided in spacious, sunny dayrooms of the Johns Hopkins Care Center on the Hopkins Bayview campus. (HBBMS)

Andrew Munster (1935-2003), right, and **Robert Spence**, opposite, made the Baltimore Regional Burn Center at Hopkins Bayview a model of its kind, treating more than 300 patients annually. Munster made extraordinary contributions to burn care, particularly in the areas of burn infection research and wound care. He wrote numerous book chapters, papers and individual books, including *Severe Burns: A Family Guide to Medical and Emotional Recovery*, published shortly before his death. He was active in dozens of professional societies, including the American Burn Association, of which he was president in 1995, and The Transplant Resource Center of Maryland, for which he was director of the Tissue Bank in 2003. Munster also served on nearly 20 state, national and international committees, presented papers extensively and received many grant awards. (HBBMS)

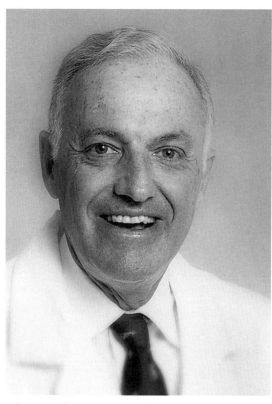

Hopkins takeover. The innovation and achievements for which the Eastern Avenue medical enclave had long been known also were given renewed impetus, resulting in some typically impressive accomplishments.

A concentration on geriatric care remained a cornerstone of the facility. Under the leadership of John R. Burton, director of the division of geriatric medicine and gerontology, FSK's fellowship program became one of the largest and most respected in the nation, and it boasted Baltimore's most extensive complement of programs for the elderly. Other facilities and programs included the Beacham Adult Day Care Center (opened in 1983 and named in honor of Edmund Beacham, the long-time chief of chronic medical care); the Beacham Ambulatory Care Center; the Physician House Call Program; and Respite Care, which provided temporary accommodations in the Lord Chronic Hospital and Nursing Facility for elderly people whose caregiving relatives required brief relief from the demands placed upon them.[64]

In 1985, the Robert Wood Johnson Foundation gave FSK a three-year grant to fund the geriatrics division's ElderCall program, which was designed to enable infirm senior citizens who lived on their own to maintain their independence. By acting as a "matchmaker" between the seniors and social service agencies, ElderCall representatives helped the elderly overcome age-related obstacles to obtaining what they needed in the way of at-home therapy, housekeeping and shopping. Within a year, the program was providing help to nearly 200 seniors. Sometimes the assistance was as simple as suggesting that an elderly woman replace her small, bedside throw rug, on which she had slipped and fallen several times, with a suction-secured bath mat.[65]

Faculty members specializing in geriatrics received prestigious fellowships and awards. Reuben Andres, clinical director of the National Institute on Aging Gerontology Research Center at FSK, received the 1986 Allied-Signal, Inc. Achievement Award in Aging, with its $30,000 cash prize. It recognized his continuous, outstanding studies in clinical gerontology and geriatric medicine. And Richard G. Bennett, a fellow in clinical geriatrics, won the 1987 Pfizer/American Geriatrics Postdoctoral Fellowship, which provided two years' salary for Bennett to conduct a study of an infection commonly found in the gastrointestinal tracts of nursing home patients who were treated with antibiotics.[66]

On other medical fronts, FSK began a two-year screening program of more than 15,000 smokers in 1987, searching for ways to combat such chronic obstructive pulmonary diseases (COPDs) as emphysema, asthma and chronic bronchitis. The screening, the largest ever conducted at the hospital, was part of a $30 million, five-year National Heart, Lung, and Blood Institute grant that was shared by 10 university medical centers. Two years later, re-

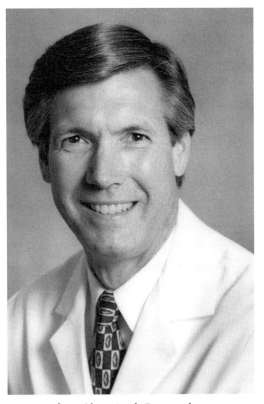

searchers at FSK's newly opened Center for Chemical Dependency were among scientists at only four U.S. facilities to conduct clinical trials to test the effectiveness and safety of a nicotine skin patch to help smokers quit. For days after the skin patch study was announced, the center was swamped with more than 2,000 telephone calls from eager prospective participants who mistakenly thought the hospital was offering a quit-smoking program, not seeking subjects for a study that required only 70 volunteers.[67]

Progress also was made on plans for building a large Asthma & Allergy Center for the Johns Hopkins School of Medicine. To make way for the five-story, 230,000-square-foot research and patient facility, the 65-year-old Bayview Asylum superintendent's residence—with its elegant French doors facing Eastern Avenue, its polished wood floors and comfortable fireplace—had to be torn down. For many years it had been the headquarters of the hospital's volunteer center, and souvenir bricks from the building were presented to director of volunteers Ann Sussman and several of her predecessors, Carolyn Cochran, Ann McDowell and Peggy Waxter (the widow of Judge Thomas Waxter, City Hospitals' staunch supporter in the 1930s). "Sometimes progress can be painful," Peterson told the volunteers, past and present, who gathered for one last tour through the house.[68]

Under the leadership of Andrew M. Munster, the Baltimore Regional Burn Center at FSK adopted a special team-treatment concept. In addition to the careful attention of its physicians, the Burn Center's patients were aided by psychologists, sociologists, vocational rehabilitation counselors, clergy,

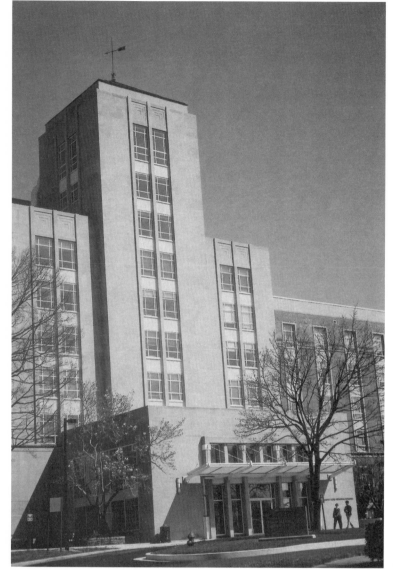

The Mason F. Lord Building, erected in 1866 and repeatedly renovated and updated, now is home to some of the finest modern laboratories on the Hopkins Bayview campus. The 138-year-old weathervane crowning its tower also signaled wind changes atop the building's original dome, which was dismantled in 1954. (JHMOCC)

home health nurses and the Burn Victims' Aid Society. This multifaceted approach helped the patients achieve not only medical recovery but emotional and professional renewal as well.[69] Proclaimed the "Best of Baltimore's Best" by Mayor Schaefer in a 1985 ceremony that included honors for Oprah Winfrey (once a local television reporter in Baltimore) and Orioles' first baseman and future Baseball Hall of Famer Eddie Murray, the Center continued its advanced work and expansion. In 1988, an eight-member team of anesthesiologists, surgeons and nurses there performed the first cultured skin graft in Maryland on a 46-year-old victim of a house fire who had sustained second- and third-degree burns over 75 percent of his body. Later that year, the center completed significant renovations that were funded in part by a $250,000 state grant.[70] In time, the center attained a 95 percent survival rate for its patients, making it one of the country's premier burn centers.[71]

In November 1988, four and a half years after Hopkins had acquired City Hospitals, a groundbreaking ceremony was held for the new $17.5 million Geriatrics Center, the first project to be launched in the multimillion-dollar Phase I Redevelopment Program for FSK. The 130,000-square-foot center would provide 190 skilled nursing facility beds, 60 chronic hospital beds, FSK's respite and adult care programs, the home care/outreach assessment team, an outpatient care center and a children's day care center. Most rooms would be semiprivate, with two patients to a room; 18 rooms would be private, and there would be six isolation rooms—quite a change from the antiquated Lord Building's arrangement of four to six patients to a room. "What we are creating here is a new national role model for a continuum of care for the elderly," John Burton told those assembled for the groundbreaking (including the residents of the Mason F. Lord Building, brought over in wheelchairs). "The elderly need a comprehensive system of care that covers the whole range of programs from ambulatory services to nursing home care. In addition, we at this Medical Center have an enormous commitment to teaching and research, and it is most unusual to have these components tied directly into long-term and other geriatric care."[72]

By the end of 1988, FSK's admissions had broken the 12,000 mark for the first time, rising from the previous year's 11,703 to 12,451. It was one of the few hospitals in Maryland to register annual increases in inpatient admissions.[73]

More advances and accolades came its way in 1989. The Division of Digestive Diseases, which annually treated more than 2,000 patients, opened a new endoscopy suite with the finest available equipment and technology for treating patients with such disorders as ulcers, colon growths and gastrointestinal bleeding. FSK's senior clinical pharmacist, Brian Katona, received a $3,500 grant from Roche Laboratories to continue his study of ways to decrease medication costs in the intensive care unit—research that already had saved the medical center $24,000 over a three-year period. FSK also opened Maryland's first four- to seven-day inpatient center for adolescent drug addicts. It had the capacity to admit young people immediately and treat them apart from adults as they began the lengthy rehabilitation process with an acute detoxification program. The leadership of scientists at The Johns Hopkins University School of Medicine's Behavioral Pharmacology Research Unit, located at FSK, led to a $10 million, five-year grant from the National Institute on Drug Abuse to develop improved ways to treat intravenous drug users as a way to prevent the spread of AIDS. The grant was unique in that it fully funded not only traditional research but a treatment facility as well.[74]

Phase I of the redevelopment project was given dramatic—indeed, explosive—punctuation on August 27, 1989, with the demolition by dynamite of the old nine-story nurses' residence, built in 1931 and more recently host to a nursing school, an HMO, a branch of the Baltimore City Department of Social Services and an assortment of offices for hospital employees.

The demise of the old structure, by then named the Community Services Center (CSC), was not devoid of sentiment. Its Art Deco design had admirers; many young nurses had trained and lived there. But by the mid-1980s, it had antiquated heating and electrical systems, no space for computer wiring, and it

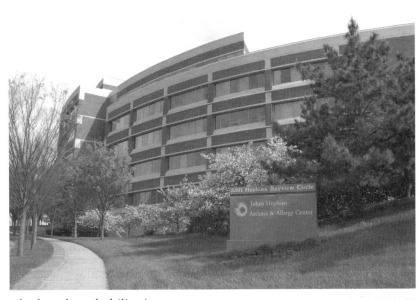

The Johns Hopkins University School of Medicine's Asthma & Allergy Center, believed to be the largest center in the nation focusing on the research and treatment of breathing disorders, opened at FSKMC in November 1989. The Triad Technology Center, which was Baltimore's first laboratory and office facility designed for the biotech and biomedical industry, had opened five months earlier. Both centers reflected the university's strong commitment to the campus. **(HBBMS)**

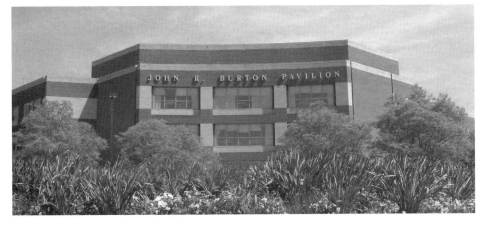

Johns Hopkins' comprehensive and highly integrated care programs for the elderly are headquartered at **the John R. Burton Pavilion** of the Johns Hopkins Bayview Care Center. The opening of the $17.5 million, 250-bed center in 1991 marked completion of Phase I of the campus' rejuvenation. It unites all of Hopkins Medicine's resources for seniors, including outpatient programs, in one, innovatively designed facility. "The entire system, from the variety of programs we offer, to the homelike, comfortable and efficient physical plant, is unique," said Burton. **(JHMOCC)**

could not be centrally air-conditioned. "It was not a user-friendly building," Bill Ward observed at the time.[75]

Ward found that the implosion method of demolition was by far the most "user-friendly"—safest, most efficient and least disruptive—means for bringing down the building, which was located near the medical center's main entrance. Controlled Demolition, Inc. (CDI) of Towson, which had an international reputation for demolishing buildings in only seconds, not the weeks or months required to knock them down using a wrecking ball, was hired to do the job. Preparations for the big blast began more than a year before the demolition date. Community residents in the immediate vicinity of the implosion were kept fully briefed; those who lived in the 12 houses closest to the site were evacuated temporarily. Parking that morning was banned on nearby streets; the city blocked traffic on Eastern Avenue; the emergency room was closed briefly (arrangements had been made to send emergency cases elsewhere, if necessary); and teams of employees directed traffic on the campus so neighborhood people could get a good view of the demolition from a safe distance. Even a motion picture crew working on "Opportunity Knocks," a comedy otherwise being filmed in Chicago starring Dana Carvey and Robert Loggia, was on hand. Because the CSC looked like a building that would be seen in the movie and suffer a similar fate, the filmmakers saw no need to pay for special effects when they could photograph them for free.[76]

VIP spectators stood on the roof of the not yet completed Asthma & Allergy Center, and hundreds of Baltimoreans gathered to watch the show. Synchronized explosions brought the building down in just six seconds, sending a billowing dust cloud high into the sky but leaving a relatively neat pile of rubble. So precise was CDI's planning and placement of the explosive devices that two trees standing only a few feet from the old building's entrance were left unscathed. Damage to the surrounding neighborhood was limited to a few window panes broken by the force of the blast.[77]

A new road would go through the site vacated by the Community Service Center, facilitating movement around a campus where more new buildings were going up than old ones were coming down. The $16 million Triad Technology Center, Baltimore's first laboratory and office facility designed for the biotech and biomedical industry, was opened two months before CDI's explosives demolished the service center. And three months after the CSC tumbled down, the Hopkins School of Medicine's Asthma & Allergy Center opened in November 1989.

The $45 million building, believed to be the largest center in the nation focusing on the research and treatment of breathing disorders, housed sophisticated basic science laboratories and patient care areas. It provided a fully integrated home for allergy and asthma programs that previously were dispersed throughout Johns Hopkins, Good Samaritan and the FSK hospitals, as well as for the Johns Hopkins Sleep Disorders Center.[78]

Scientists moving into the new center already were obtaining more than $8 million in research grants annually and were credited with developing techniques to evaluate the effectiveness of allergy shots, provide immunity against insect-sting allergy and help people with asthma breathe. The center's primary focus was to be on determining the mechanism of asthma and devising new treatments for allergies and breathing disorders. At the dedication ceremony, Claude Lenfant, director of the National Heart, Lung, and Blood Institute, praised the center's opening as "a major step in the search for the prevention and cure for asthma."[79]

Following the ceremonies, as the celebrants were toasting the new center, disaster struck the 25-year-old AA Building, in which Peterson and other FSK administrators had their offices. Pipes in the ceiling burst and water cascaded down into the offices, flooding them up to several inches in depth. Peterson, Ward, Grabill and Reitz—all in black-tie finery at the Asthma Center—were summoned by facilities workers to the waterlogged offices.

"Here we were with this grand, new, beautiful building opening up, and across the way we were falling apart," recalls Susan Davis, the long-time public affairs chief at the hospital, with a rueful chuckle.

With the end of fiscal 1990 in sight, Peterson's team had recorded five straight years of positive cash flow. Their achievement opened the door to the debt financing markets, enabling FSK to sell tax-exempt revenue bonds through the Maryland Health and Higher Education Facilities Authority (MHHEFA) to finance more new buildings that would ensure the revitalization of the campus. Surveying his soggy office, Peterson knew only too well how much they needed the money.

A miracle of medical center rejuvenation had begun on Eastern Avenue, but bringing it to fruition would not be easy.

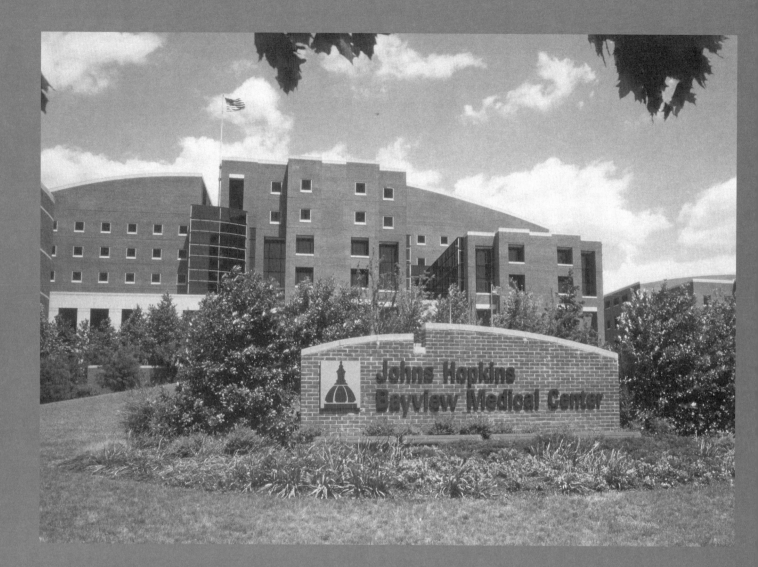

The Francis Scott Key Pavilion today. (HBBMS)

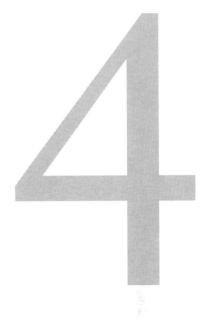

"...nothing short
of miraculous..."

AS FORWARD-LOOKING AS WERE THE PHASE I REVITALIZATION plans for the Francis Scott Key Medical Center, a sense of the institution's illustrious, yet at times troubled past never was far from the thoughts of the people working to ensure its future.

Sometimes reminders of that past resurfaced in bizarre ways. During the construction of the new comprehensive geriatrics center in the fall of 1989, workers using a backhoe to grade land around its foundation unearthed more than rocks, roots and dirt. They found unmarked graves.[1]

Five skeletons, determined by city archaeologists to be 100 years old, were discovered. They dated from the days when the hospital was known as the Bay View Asylum. Since no records could be found indicating that asylum patients or residents ever were buried on the grounds, the identities of the skeletons remained mysterious. After the archaeologists completed a week-long excavation of the burial site without uncovering additional telltale artifacts, the skeletons quietly were transferred to a private cemetery elsewhere, and construction of the geriatrics center proceeded.[2]

Bill Ward told *Community News*, a FSK publication distributed in the neighborhoods surrounding the hospital, that while finding the skeletons definitely was "unusual," the project otherwise was "routine." The building going up, however, was anything but conventional.

"The design is such that it draws patients out of their rooms and into the spacious, sunny dayrooms," Ward explained enthusiastically. "This will give the facility a greater sense of hominess and community. The design also will be convenient and efficient for staff—each resident will be only a short walk away." John Burton, director of geriatrics, praised the new center's design as an ideal match between form and function. "The entire system, from the variety of programs we offer, to the homelike, comfortable and efficient physical plant, is unique," he said.[3]

Construction of the innovative geriatrics center, as well as the plans being drawn up for even more advanced facilities, were fueled by FSK's continuing financial success. Fiscal year 1990 ended with FSK recording a $3.2 million profit, marking the fifth year in a row that revenues exceeded expenses. Since 1986, the medical center had averaged $3.5 million in annual profits, just the

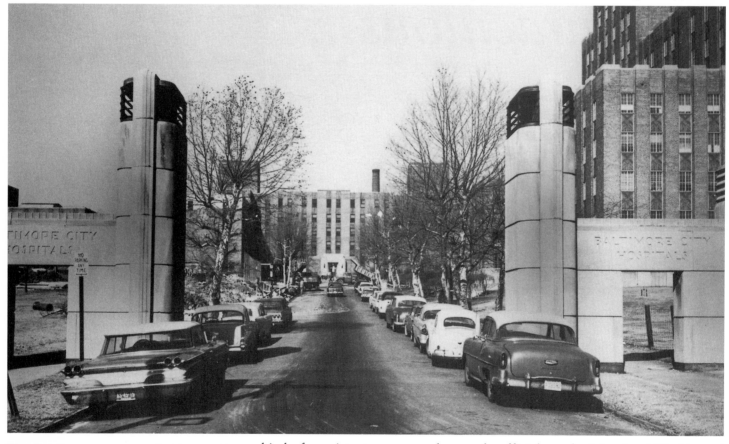

The Art Deco entrance to Baltimore City Hospitals greeted visitors in the 1960s as they approached the A Building, completed in 1935. Today it frames the Francis Scott Key Pavilion of Hopkins Bayview, opened in 1994. (Above, HBBMS; opposite, JHMOCC)

kind of consistent successes that made officials at the Maryland Health and Higher Educational Facilities Authority (MHHEFA) confident that issuing revenue bonds to fund more construction at FSK was a sound investment.[4]

By the fall of 1990, planning already was moving forward aggressively on Phase II of the redevelopment program. MHHEFA began selling bonds to garner $100 million in funds to pay for a new, 275,000-square-foot inpatient facility, renovations to the Mason F. Lord Building, and repayment of some of the interim financing for Phase I of the revitalization.[5] "The redevelopment of this medical center is an enormous effort," Ward told *Community News*. "The work has been made easier because of the cooperation, understanding and support we've had from our staff, the doctors, the patients and the community. Everyone has a stake in this project, and everyone is working to make sure it succeeds."[6]

Hard-hatted construction workers and lumbering bulldozers became familiar sights on the FSK campus while the impressive work of its existing programs and personnel continued.

Surgical procedures offered by the new burn treatment program included scar revision, skin resurfacing, contracture release, reconstruction of lost and damaged parts, repigmentation and hand surgery. Health care professionals from several disciplines, including physical therapy, occupational therapy and social work, as well as a psychologist and a nurse coordinator, were given

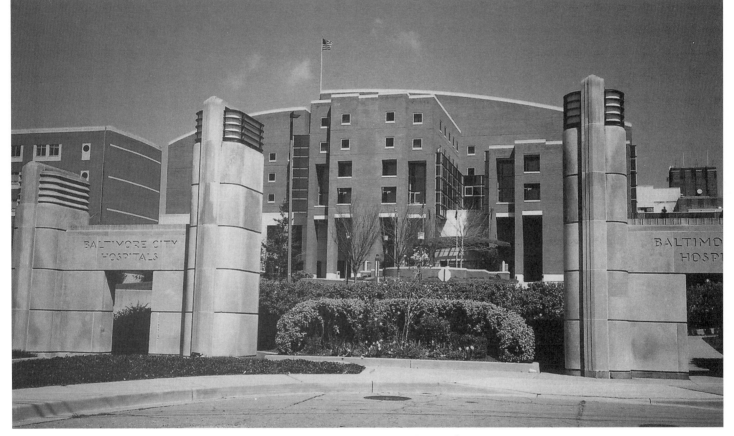

major roles to play in the program—as was a corrective cosmetician, who could show patients how to use makeup to hide some of the skin damage caused by burns. The new program, Robert J. Spence said at the time, served patients more effectively because they were provided with "a planned structure throughout the entire rehabilitation process."[7]

In September 1990, the Baltimore Regional Burn Center opened a new Center for Burn Reconstruction, offering a comprehensive program that integrated reconstruction and aesthetic surgery with various support services, making it one of the few centers in the country that linked such support efforts to an acute burn center. Under the direction of Spence, chief of plastic surgery at FSK and co-director of the Burn Center, the new program provided

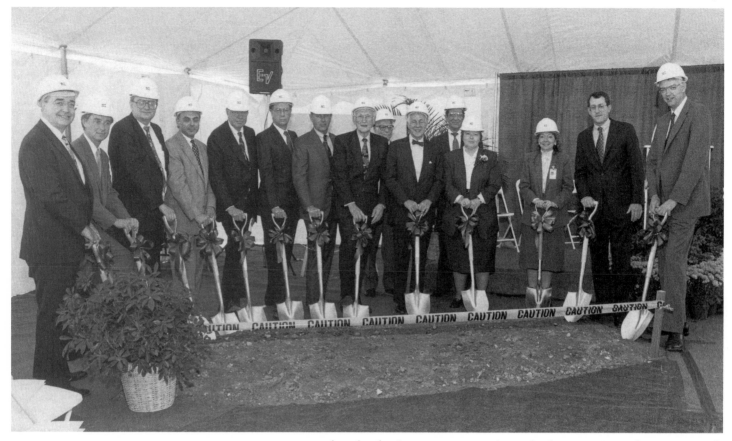

Charles Benton, former director of finance for Baltimore city under Mayor Schaefer, is the central figure in this line-up of ceremonial ground-breakers for the Francis Scott Key Pavilion in 1991. Benton was the tough but willing bargainer during lengthy negotiations between the city and Johns Hopkins over the acquisition of City Hospitals. From left, **Robert Shaff** of Whiting-Turner contractors; trustee **Francis Knott; David Beard** of RTKL architects; **Michael Johns,** dean of the Hopkins School of Medicine; **Robert Heyssel,** president of The Johns Hopkins Hospital; **Philip Zieve; Chester Schmidt Jr.;** Benton; trustee **Walter Sondheim Jr.;** trustee chairman **Robert D.H. Harvey; Gardner Smith;** nursing director **Carol Ball; Judy Reitz,** Bayview's vice president for nursing; **Ronald R. Peterson,** Bayview's president; **William Ward,** Bayview's vice president for operations. (HBBMS)

a structured and cohesive treatment regimen for burn patients, beginning with their admission.

Former Burn Center patients also played a central role in that rehabilitation process, returning once a week as part of an informal support program. They would meet with current patients and provide not only sympathy but inspiration. Andrew Munster called the former patients' activities "critical" to the recovery of the present patients. "Even professionals—nurses, doctors, counselors—cannot do what these people can do for our patients," he told *Community News.*[8]

The Burn Center (which would mark its 25th anniversary in 1993) continued to receive substantial financial support from the local Kiwanis club, as well as from the Metropolitan Fire Fighters Burn Center Fund, sponsored by firefighters and officers from Baltimore City, Annapolis, Baltimore-Washington International Airport, and Baltimore, Anne Arundel and Howard counties; and from the Baltimore Regional Burn Center Foundation. The foundation funded burn prevention programs and a special "re-entry" educational program for schoolchildren who had missed classes because of hospitalization for burns; and a free summertime Burn Camp for youngsters recovering from burns.[9]

Other new centers opened at FSK to address a variety of medical and community issues. The Johns Hopkins Obesity Center established a new treatment program to provide comprehensive, medically supervised weightloss and management options ranging from behavior modification to gastric surgery; and the Johns Hopkins School of Hygiene and Public Health and the School of Medicine joined forces with FSK to open the Center for Occupational and Environmental Health on the FSK campus.[10]

Directed by James R. Nethercott, the new occupational health center combined faculty expertise in occupational medicine, pulmonary medicine, toxicology, dermatology, epidemiology, Lyme disease and follow-up care for injuries. Its focus was on providing public health services and medical care to private industry, state and federal government agencies and individuals through programs in public health practice and clinical occupational medicine. It offered medical surveillance and biological monitoring, health promotion programs, executive health assessment programs, industrial hygiene assessments and health hazard evaluations. The center's clinical occupational medicine program conducted third-party medical assessments, acute injury and fume intoxication management, and secondary and tertiary consultative services.[11]

In another collaboration, the Maryland Department of Health and Mental Hygiene joined federal agencies to award grants totaling $800,000 to FSK for creation of the Center for Addiction and Pregnancy (CAP). Providing comprehensive care for pregnant women addicted to heroin, cocaine, alcohol and other drugs, CAP sought to help the women end their addiction and thereby reduce the number and severity of obstetric complications—including HIV

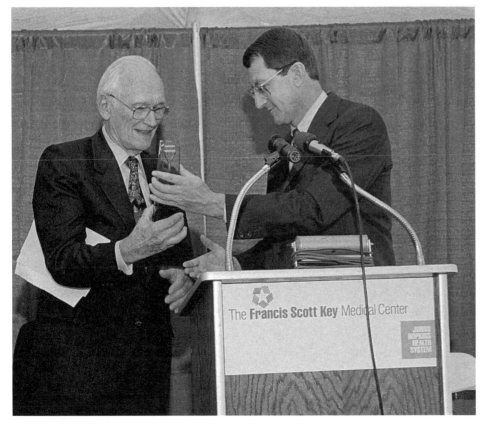

A gift is presented to **Charles Benton,** former Baltimore finance director, left, by **Ronald Peterson,** his former employee (as Johns Hopkins' executive director of Baltimore City Hospitals, working under contract to the city) at groundbreaking for the Francis Scott Key Pavilion in 1991. As secretary of the Maryland Department of Budget and Fiscal Planning under Governor Schaefer at the time of this groundbreaking, Benton called the revitalization of the Eastern Avenue campus "nothing short of miraculous." (HBBMS)

Reminders of the past are everywhere on the Eastern Avenue campus; some were found beneath it. In 1989, workers grading land for FSKMC's new comprehensive geriatrics center found five skeletons, which archeologists determined were a century old. Twenty-eight years earlier, in 1961, another group of skeletons dating from the Bay View Asylum era were uncovered in what was believed to have been the institution's paupers' burial ground. (Photo by William K. Mortimer, ©1961 *The Baltimore Sun.* Used by permission.)

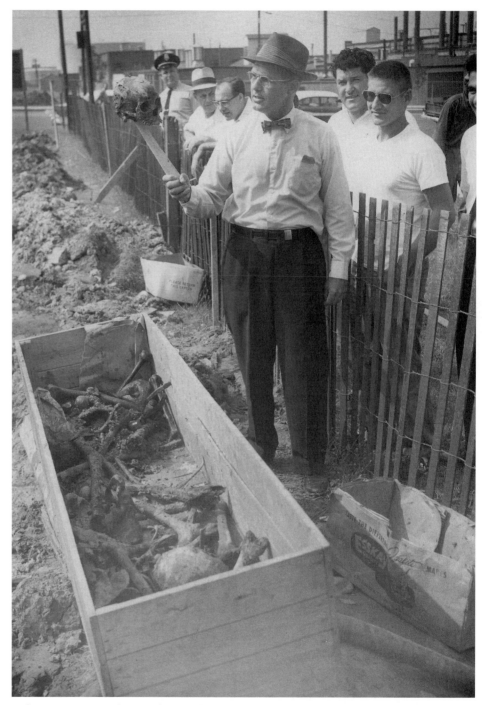

infection—imperiling infants of mothers who no longer were abusing illegal drugs or alcohol. The program also aimed to ensure initial and long-term pediatric assessment for these babies.[12]

"We are dealing with the suppressed, covered-up sense of commitment that most mothers have for their children," George R. Huggins, chairman of FSK's Department of Obstetrics and Gynecology and head of the new center, told a press briefing when the creation of CAP was announced.[13] "And if we can get their heads clear enough so that the maternal instinct can wake again, we have something powerful going for us that doesn't happen in other drug treatment programs."

Within six months of CAP's opening in May 1991, Huggins reported an encouraging rise in the birth weight of infants born to mothers in the program, and a dramatic reduction in the number of their newborns requiring admission to the hospital's neonatal intensive care unit—saving more than $224,910 in hospital costs. After a year in operation, CAP estimated that the savings had risen another $151,350, for a total of $376,260.[14]

Honors also continued to come to FSK faculty and staff. In October 1990, J. Ken Waters, assistant director of the hospital's pharmacy, received the Paul G. Pierpaoli Award from the Connecticut Society of Hospital Pharmacists; and Robert J. Gregerman, chief of the FSK's division of endocrinology, received the Clinical Gerontology Research Award from the American Aging Association.[15]

Recognition even came to the extensive efforts of southeast Baltimore community volunteers to provide services and amenities to FSK patients. As part of his "Daily Point of Light" program, President George H.W. Bush saluted the 30 members of FSK's Thursday Volunteer Group in May 1991 for spending more than 100,000 hours over a 15-year period to entertain and assist residents at the Mason F. Lord Chronic Hospital and Nursing Facility. The Thursday Volunteers, local residents who all were over 65 years of age, provided a weekly band concert featuring retired professional musicians, plus refreshments, to the elderly patients; transported them to religious services each Sunday; and offered comfort and support to those without immediate family members.[16]

Less than a month after the presidential kudos for the volunteers at the chronic hospital and nursing facility, the patients they served received a brand new home when the $17.5 million Johns Hopkins Geriatrics Center opened on June 6, 1991. The six-story, 250-bed, red brick center became the hub of Hopkins Geriatrics, a new systemwide initiative uniting all of Hopkins Medicine's resources for seniors in one facility.[17]

The Hopkins Geriatrics initiative provided an extensive core of services,

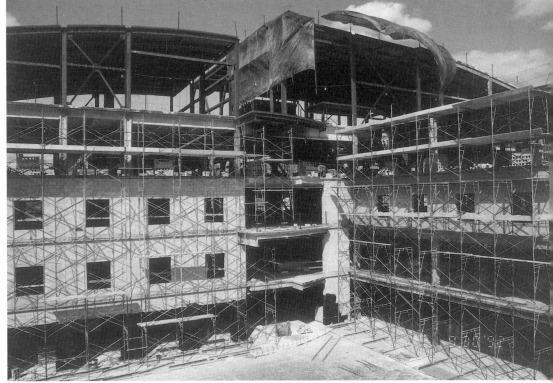

The **Francis Scott Key Pavilion** under construction. (HBBMS)

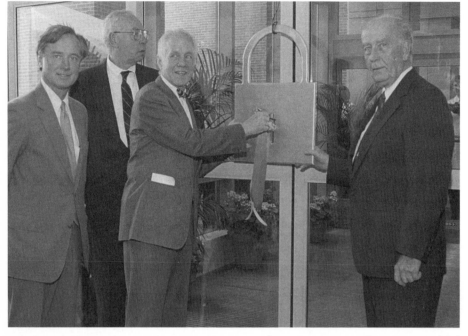

Governor William Donald Schaefer (right) was amazed at the transformation of the old City Hospitals and lavished praise—some of it rueful—on the people who accomplished it. A decade after the transfer, Schaefer told the crowd at dedication ceremonies for the Francis Scott Key Pavilion at the Johns Hopkins Bayview Medical Center: "In the first year, they broke even.... In the second year ... [they] made a profit. And the third year, I knew we'd made a bad deal!" Shown along with Schaefer using a large ceremonial key to open the Key Pavilion are (from left) trustee **Francis Knott; Robert Heyssel,** president of The Johns Hopkins Hospital, and Bayview board of trustees chairman **Robert D.H. Harvey.** (HBBMS)

including inpatient units for chronic, skilled and rehabilitation care. Complementing these services were outpatient programs for adult day care, geriatric assessment, incontinence and physician house calls. "The care programs we have developed for elderly persons at Francis Scott Key are designed to be comprehensive and highly integrated," John Burton said at the time of the opening of the Geriatrics Center. (Ten years later, it would be named for him).[18]

"Very elderly patients, who are highly dependent in many of their daily needs, require such a system, which allows them to move from one program to another as their needs change. Our goal is to provide the most appropriate care, which will emphasize independence, compassion and human dignity for each individual."

Each floor of the center's residential areas had rooms situated in three "residential clusters," designed to encourage the residents to socialize with their neighbors. The clusters converged on large, airy community rooms that were bathed in natural light coming from huge picture windows offering spectacular views of the Baltimore skyline. Regular windows on each floor were set low in the walls so residents in wheelchairs could take advantage of the view.

An acute geriatrics unit (AGU) was created in the main hospital to restore the health and enhance the independence of frail, elderly patients, many of whom still lived at home or in nursing facilities. The AGU, directed by Burton and William Greenough, from the Division of Geriatric Medicine and Gerontology at the Hopkins School of Medicine, emphasized not only excellent patient care but the education of future physicians and nurses in geriatrics. The AGU's success in treating patients with chronic conditions prompted a steady stream of inquiries from other hospitals around the country, who themselves sought to learn from Hopkins' geriatrics expertise, which now was centered at FSK.[19]

The dedication of the Geriatrics Center was immensely satisfying for Peterson and his colleagues, marking as it did the official completion of Phase I of their redevelopment master plan. They had achieved an astounding turnaround in just seven years, and the pride in their accomplishment was palpable. Peterson, whose usually dignified demeanor and penchant for conservative, dark blue suits disguised an antic sense of humor, even permitted himself a brief public display of his comedic abilities, much to the astonishment and delight of those present.

The keynote speaker for the event was to be U.S. Surgeon General Antonia C. Novello, a graduate of the Johns Hopkins School of Hygiene and Public Health and the first woman and first Hispanic to be appointed Surgeon General. A busy public official who was also unfamiliar with the roads leading to FSK, she was reported to be running far behind schedule and would be late for the ceremony. Peterson, amused by the fact that Novello was the sister-in-law of comedian Don Novello, creator of "Father Guido Sarducci," a favorite character of his on "Saturday Night Live," decided that he should "explain" the reasons for the guest of honor's tardiness with a purported "Mailgram" from Father Guido.

"I'm not going to vouch for its legitimacy," Peterson said with a deadpan, "but let me read it to you." Then, expertly imitating Don Novello's mock Italian accent, Peterson proceeded, to increasingly loud laughs:

"Dear Mr. Peteda-sone:

"I'm-a so sorry to hav-a ta be the one to inform you that my sista-in-law, the Surgeon General, has-a propensity to be-a little late from-a time-a to time. Bu' donna worry. She don't mean nothin' by it. You just see, Mr. Peteda-sone, very important-a people, they sometimes-a get-a booked back-a-to-back. She be there soon—but not-a yet.

"Keep-a da faith, keep-a da faith."

"That's signed, 'His Irreverence, Father Guido Sarducci'," Peterson concluded, to much applause following the laughter. Later, when Baltimore Mayor Kurt Schmoke took the podium to acknowledge the arrival of Novello, he quipped, "I did want to welcome Dr. Novello, but Ron, you did such a wonderful job, I'm not going to even touch that right now."[20]

Robert Heyssel, whom Peterson introduced as "the individual who gave me the opportunity to come to Baltimore City Hospitals in 1982, and at the same time was the guy who had the wisdom to... let me do my own thing out here," surveyed the impressive new geriatrics center and other evidence of the vitality on the FSK campus with satisfaction and a touch of awe. His gamble in acquiring City Hospitals clearly was paying off, as was his faith in Peterson— who, he noted wryly, probably didn't think "it was such a privilege when I asked him to come out here in 1982.

"I look around a little amazed... at what has been accomplished," Heyssel said. As for Peterson and his team, Heyssel added: "I left him alone because he's smarter than I am, and he did everything we expected, plus. And I'm sure he will continue to, and I hope you'll all come back in about two years, when we dedicate what will then be the acute care facility on this campus.... I think we will be coming back and back and back to this site to see both good things

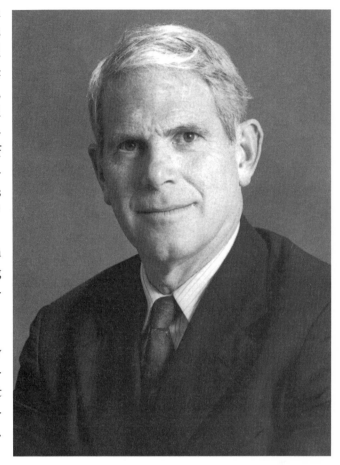

John R. Burton, Mason F. Lord Professor of Medicine, was for more than 20 years the driving force in the development of geriatrics at Johns Hopkins Bayview. He was a nationally prominent figure in the field as director of the Division of Geriatric Medicine and Gerontology in The Johns Hopkins University School of Medicine, where he initiated innovative clinical, training and research programs. Dedicated to teaching and committed to compassionate patient care, Burton continues his busy clinical practice and leads a nationwide effort to enhance geriatric education in medical schools. **(HBBMS)**

Louis Kavoussi, left, and Lloyd Ratner prepare to perform the first laparoscopic kidney transplant in November 1995. Hopkins Bayview has been in the forefront of developing minimally invasive surgical techniques. (HBBMS)

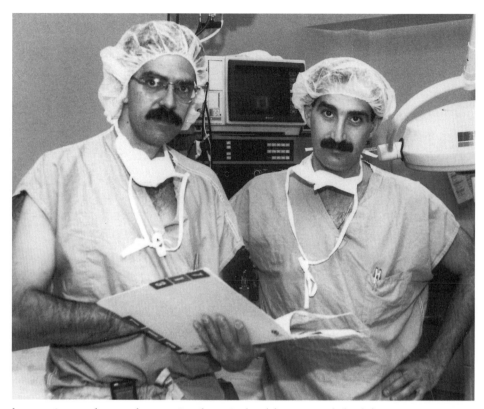

happening and more happening here in health care and the life sciences."[21]

Only four months later, in October 1991, many of the same Hopkins and city officials gathered on the exact spot where the ceremony officially transferring City Hospitals to Hopkins ownership had taken place in 1984, to break ground for the new 275,000-square-foot, 221-bed acute care tower Heyssel had mentioned.[22] It would be funded primarily through revenue bonds, but also from the proceeds of a $3.5 million fund-raising effort, the first capital campaign ever undertaken for the FSK Medical Center.[23]

The chairman of the hospital's board of trustees, Robert D.H. Harvey, told the gathering that when Johns Hopkins "the man" had penned his will nearly 120 years earlier, he really "had no idea" the scope of the changes in medicine that would be wrought by the hospital his benefaction would found. Harvey predicted that over the next 15 years, there was "not only the opportunity for, but the probability of, changes in the future at the Francis Scott Key campus "way beyond the change that has occurred to the Johns Hopkins Hospital in a full 100 years." The pioneering work already accomplished at FSK—in its burn center, its gastrointestinal pain management program, its kidney dialysis initiative—were "just ripples on the ocean's surface," Harvey said. "Gigantic tidal changes" in medical service at the center lay ahead.[24]

The guest speaker for the acute patient care tower groundbreaking was none other than Charles Benton, the former city finance chief who had proven such a tough bargainer in the lengthy negotiations over the transfer of City Hospitals to Hopkins' control. When Baltimore's Mayor Schaefer had become

Maryland's governor in 1987, Benton went with him to Annapolis, becoming secretary of the Maryland Department of Budget and Fiscal Planning. Ron Peterson, introducing Benton, observed that he and the mayor "could easily have decided to sell City Hospitals to the highest bidder—but, of course, we all know... my boss, Heyssel, was not the highest bidder." Benton laughed along with the rest of the audience. Peterson said he hoped Benton would agree that the transaction that was concluded between Hopkins and the city had "served all parties very well, and I hope that is true for the citizens whom we serve."[25]

Benton, in humorously recounting the drawn-out bargaining over City Hospitals' fate, said he viewed the acute patient tower's groundbreaking ceremony "with a great deal of personal satisfaction," as well as a "vindication" of the city's decision to divest itself of City Hospitals. "Now as I look around and see the vast improvements that have already been made and those in the planning stage, I would say that this transformation is nothing short of miraculous," he said.[26]

Peterson also called upon Philip Zieve, the veteran chief of medicine, to speak. Zieve, with his nearly 35 years of experience on Eastern Avenue, observed that despite the wonderful prospects of improved treatment facilities in the new patient tower, "it... [is] not buildings that define this institution. Buildings are built and they crumble. And it's not people that define the institution, because they, too, are built and crumble. It is the mission of the place. It's what we stand for. And what we stand for is the compassionate care of the sick."[27]

That compassionate care increasingly extended beyond the walls of FSK's inpatient facilities.

The medical center operated several outpatient clinics whose physicians essentially served as family doctors to hundreds of Southeast Baltimore residents. The center's Ambulatory Services Department included medical, surgical and Ob/Gyn clinics, all staffed by faculty from the Johns Hopkins School of Medicine. Carol Ball, the director of nursing and head of the ambulatory services and clinical program, explained to Community News, "Clinic patients choose a doctor and use him or her in just the same way they would a doctor at an independent office. The only difference is, they visit the doctor here at the Medical Center."[28]

The medical center offered treatment from nearly 50 physicians in a wide range of specialties: general internal medicine, neurology, endocrinology, dermatology, hematology and other disciplines. The Ob/Gyn clinic provided care ranging from routine gynecological checkups and Pap tests to amniocentesis, ultrasonography, care of high-risk pregnancies and infertility treatments. The surgery clinic, many of whose patients were referred there by doctors in the medical and Ob/Gyn clinics, offered specialists in orthopedics, ophthalmology, otolaryngology, plastic surgery, burns, urology and neurologic and general surgery.[29]

Hopkins geriatrics also offered a wide range of outpatient and outreach services based at FSK. The Geriatric Assessment Center's doctors, nurses and social workers conducted a comprehensive evaluation of a patient's physical, mental, functional and housing status and prepared a profile report that recommended future action to the patient, the patient's family and physician. The continence clinic addressed a prevalent but distressing problem afflicting the elderly, loss of bladder control. After a thorough medical examination, doctors using biofeedback techniques and recommending specific exercises often could help patients attain significant improvement in urinary continence.

Geriatrics physicians in the Elder House Call program employed the old-fashioned, most cost-efficient means of treatment; they made house calls. A patient coordinator would help individuals arrange various services, including home X-rays, blood tests, electrocardiograph readings and prescription deliveries. The Beacham Ambulatory Care Center provided a complete range of medical services to patients in nearby neighborhoods, and the Beacham Adult Day Care Center offered an excellent daytime alternative to nursing home placement. Another program, Senior Companions, employed low-income elderly people who were trained by the Baltimore City Health Department to provide such simple, yet invaluable services as light housekeeping and reading to homebound neighbors.[30]

In addition, Hopkins Geriatrics provided other services designed to meet the special needs of the elderly, including dementia/Alzheimer's programs; geriatric neurology assessments and evaluations of such neurological problems as memory loss; psychogeriatrics, which provided psychiatric consultations and treatments for the elderly and their caregivers; and the functional status laboratory at The Johns Hopkins Hospital, which tested and evaluated elderly patients for problems such as limited stamina, vision and balance problems and propensity to fall. The Hopkins Home Care service provided such specialties as private duty nursing, home health aide assistance, and introductions to appropriate community services.[31]

"Preventing hospitalization is what Hopkins geriatrics is all about," John Burton told *Community News*. His innovative Elder House Call program was spotlighted in a National Public Radio feature report.[32]

Under Gayle Johnson Adams' energetic leadership, FSK also launched many "health awareness" and community outreach programs. Its South East Emergency Needs Network (SEENN) operated a prescription assistance fund for the needy, in addition to its emergency food closet. Each month, FSK health care professionals also offered free blood pressure screenings at community sites, and arranged to do other screenings to assess weight, lung function and medication. In conjunction with the Greater Baltimore Committee and the Baltimore City Public Schools, FSK sponsored a partnership program with a number of elementary, middle and high schools in the community, enabling students to learn about health care and career opportunities in the field.

Additional educational programs included FRESH (Food Re-education for Elementary School Health), an effort to reduce the risk of future heart disease by teaching children how to lower their cholesterol and blood pressure through better eating and exercise; the Emergency Nurses C.A.R.E. Program, which taught high school students about the consequences of drinking and driving; the Safe Sitter program, a 13-hour course designed for 11- to 14-year-olds on first aid, life-saving techniques and the responsibilities and ethics of safe babysitting; and the Center for Breastfeeding, providing support, assistance and helpful information to young mothers. Project Independence provided training and work experience opportunities to help participants obtain entry-level jobs.

Along with its week-long summer camp for former burn patients ages 8 to 16, its School Re-Entry Program, and its Burn Survivors Support Group, FSK also joined with the American Lung Association to co-sponsor "Camp Superkids," a week-long summer camp for children with asthma and other respiratory illnesses.[33]

Within the medical center, the Johns Hopkins AIDS Service opened a 16-bed post-acute AIDS unit in July 1993, designed to serve people with AIDS who required long-term care and services that were less intensive than what was offered in the acute hospital. Given the thousands of AIDS cases in Baltimore city and the thousands of city residents who were infected with HIV but not yet suffering from AIDS, "the need for alternatives to hospital care" was growing rapidly, explained Richard E. Chaisson, director of FSK's AIDS unit and of the AIDS Service at The Johns Hopkins Hospital.[34]

The post-acute AIDS unit was the first at FSK to employ a medical service delivery model called patient-focused care, in which the patient was placed at the center of all health care activity, with emphasis on providing service with maximum efficiency.

Under patient-focused care, both the services to the patient and the unit's operation were enhanced by cross-training the staff, so that employees could handle a broader range of patient care functions and provide up to 90 percent of the services their patients needed. For example, nurses and other professionals learned how to administer respiratory treatment and electrocardiograms. Many support and ancillary operations were decentralized in order to locate services for the patient's convenience, not the providers'. For example, X-ray equipment was brought to the patient, instead of the patient being taken to an X-ray unit, reducing scheduling time and transportation needs. Improved information systems and establishment of practice guidelines helped streamline the service delivery process.[35]

Physicians, nurses, dietitians, social workers, respiratory therapists and mental health counselors in the new AIDS unit provided patients with continued health care following an acute hospital stay. Patients also received rehabilitative services, including physical and occupational therapy.[36]

Another personnel initiative launched at FSK was dubbed "Quality Service," with intradepartmental teams of employees established to collaborate with their counterparts in other departments to identify and eliminate impediments to efficient, friendly, convenient and prompt service to patients and their families.[37] "Many hospitals provide the same clinical services," Judy Reitz told *Keynotes* early in 1993. "The difference is in how they provide them. That's where Quality Service can have a great impact."[38]

In recognition of Reitz's role in fostering the adoption of quality management and service excellence initiatives, Peterson promoted her in November 1993 to the position of executive vice president and chief operating officer for FSK.

The improved service efforts paid off not only with better customer satisfaction results on periodic patient surveys, but in the steadily rising number of clinic visits, admissions and surgical procedures at FSK. From 41,903 clinic visits in 1993, the number rose to 47,852 in 1995; admissions went up from 13,735 to 15,378 during the same period, and surgical procedures rose from 5,219 to 5,881.[39]

Those patient increases also were reflected in FSK's revenue figures. The medical center reported a $3.7 million profit on $157 million in revenues in 1993, up from a $2 million profit in 1992. "Excesses of revenue over expenses" continued in the $3 million range through 1995.[40]

Five months after opening its post-acute AIDS unit, FSK announced the launch of a unique and comprehensive treatment and prevention program for people suffering from kidney stones. The new Stone Center, opened in January 1994, was the only one in Maryland to link state-of-the-art diagnostic and treatment methods and an extensive prevention program.[41]

Directed by Louis Kavoussi, chief of the Department of Urology, and David Spector, co-director of the Department of Nephrology, the Stone Center combined the fields of urology, radiology and nephrology to treat all types of kidney stones: calcium, uric acid, infection and cystine. Among the latest innovative treatment procedures the center provided was lithotripsy, in which a computerized, ultrasound wave was directed toward the kidney stones. The ultrasound wave shattered or pulverized the stones; the fragments then were passed through the urinary tract.[42]

Creating the Stone Center at FSK made sense, given Maryland's location on the northern tip of what physicians had come to call the "stone belt," the southeast portion of the United States where the highest incidence of kidney stones occurs. Kidney stones, a malady whose history can be traced to ancient times, are hard, crystalline substances made of salt and minerals found in the urine. The ultimate causes of kidney stones remain somewhat mysterious, but hot, humid climate seems to be a factor—and summertime weather in Maryland fits that bill. Besides becoming dehydrated in such a climate, people tend to absorb more vitamin D from the sun, and increased vitamin D causes an increased rate of absorption of calcium.[43]

It was also under the direction of Kavoussi, head of the Center for Minimally Invasive Surgery at FSK, that surgeons there became the first in the country to use a robotic arm, the Automated Endoscopic Systems for Optimal Positioning (AESOP), as a surgical assistant to remove a gallbladder and perform a tubal ligation, a bladder suspension and a high ligation of a left internal spermatic vein, all in one day. In all of the operations, Kavoussi and his colleagues could see the internal organs with the aid of a laparoscope, a lighted telescope AESOP inserted into the patients via dime-size incisions, and doctors performed the surgery though they were not right beside the patient.[44]

"AESOP was rock-steady in positioning and holding a tiny camera," Kavoussi said following the surgeries. "But the most exciting element of the procedure is the ability to use remote control." Kavoussi then was one of only a few researchers in the country to establish a remote-control surgical system, called telepresence surgery, that enabled surgeons to use robots to perform surgery on patients from a room adjacent to the actual OR.[45]

"Robots and telepresence surgery will not dehumanize medicine," Kavoussi said. "These remarkable changes in medicine are fueled by what patients want. They don't want surgery to hurt, they don't want it to interrupt their lifestyle for long periods of time. Robotics will enhance the procedures we do now."[46]

Fueling the development of such innovative procedures on the FSK campus were two factors in which it had an edge over the increasingly crowded North Broadway site of The Johns Hopkins Hospital: space and a lower threshold for financial returns.

"Kavoussi was one of the junior faculty guys [at Hopkins] who came on [to FSK] because he wasn't able to get access to resources" at Hopkins Hospital, says Ken Grabill.[47]

"In the eight years that I was assistant budget director at Broadway, there were, every year, programs that didn't meet our financial test" at Hopkins Hospital and thus were not approved there, Grabill says. "In my first weeks here, in September of '82, I ran into a lot of those," he recalls with a laugh. "You had space [here] that... needed to be put to a medical use... and you had pieces and parts of the Hopkins family regularly doing start-up sort of activities, a farm club kind of analogy."[48]

The clinical start-ups at FSK would not have brought in sufficient revenue at Hopkins in competition with established programs there that already were appropriately profitable, Grabill explains, noting, "Back there [on Broadway], breaking even wasn't good enough." But at FSK, a break-even program had a very desirable impact on the bottom line.

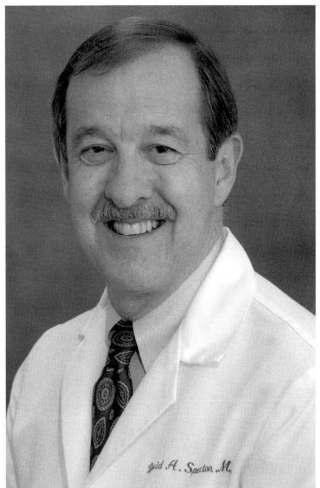

David A. Spector served as chief of nephrology from 1995 to 1999. He launched the nephrology fellowship program in 1978 and has been its director ever since. His efforts to preserve the history of Hopkins Bayview and its predecessor institutions led to the creation of an extensive archive in the Harrison Library. (HBBMS)

Kavoussi was an example of the sort of rising star in the Hopkins firmament who was given space and resources at FSK, Grabill says, then did "all sorts of fabulous activities, various minimally invasive surgeries... all sorts of developments on the research side... [and] a lot of applications in the clinical practice," improved the services, increased patient volumes, and ultimately ended up concentrating most of his efforts back on Broadway, opening up space for a new "high-flying junior faculty person" to go to Eastern Avenue to shine.[49]

The shining work at the Francis Scott Key Medical Center and its decade of profitable operations earned it something that initially had been deemed too precious to bestow: The Hopkins name.

With the approaching dedication of the acute care patient tower, the boards of the Francis Scott Key Medical Center and its parent board of the Johns Hopkins Health System decided in January 1994 to rename the facility the "Johns Hopkins Bayview Medical Center," effective the following April, in recognition of what Peterson proudly and accurately described as a "successfully completed... major redevelopment and image transformation" there.[50]

"While the new name conveys the prominent brand name of our parent, it also incorporates the unique identifier, Bayview, which has applied to this campus, on and off, since the 1860s," Peterson told the audience at the patient tower's dedication ceremony on April 26, 1994, just three months shy of the tenth anniversary of the Hopkins acquisition of City Hospitals. He added that although the medical center's name was being changed "with a sense of pride and accomplishment," the new patient tower was being christened the "Francis Scott Key Pavilion," so as to perpetuate the last decade of this institution's 221-year history.

"Many of us who have worked here during the last 10 years certainly are proud of what we've been able to accomplish under the auspices of Francis Scott Key, so there's a strong desire to utilize the Francis Scott Key name," he explained.[51]

Applying the Hopkins name to the medical center, however, emphasized "its prominence in the Johns Hopkins family of medical institutions" and would "convey effectively that Hopkins medicine is practiced here by a medical staff that is largely full-time faculty of The Johns Hopkins University School of Medicine," Peterson later wrote in *Community News*.[52]

Peterson described the Francis Scott Key Pavilion as "the crown jewel" of the six-year, two-phase, $100 million redevelopment program for the medical center—a "centerpiece" that, at a final cost of $60 million ($1 million less than originally estimated in 1991) was "a pretty cost-effective" construction project.[53]

The six-story building was configured in an L shape around the existing acute care hospital and topped with a distinctive arching roof that could be seen for miles. It contained 221 acute hospital beds (31 more than the 190 initially planned), with 40 percent of them in private rooms and 60 percent in semiprivate rooms—a considerable improvement over the 40 percent of beds in the old acute care complex that were still four to a room.[54]

In addition to providing a new home for the Burn Center, the Pavilion also housed a new, 17-bed acute geriatrics unit (AGU), more than doubling the capacity of the original, eight-bed AGU opened in 1991; an emergency department and trauma center that increased the space for these facilities by 50 percent; and a new 31-bed neurosciences unit, developed by a multidisciplinary team of clinicians for patients under treatment for stroke, brain tumors, spinal diseases, epilepsy and other neurological problems, as well as patients with carotid artery disease who require surgical opening of the vessels. A new imaging center provided for round-the-clock operation of the Pavilion's X-ray, CT scanning, nuclear medicine, and ultrasound and magnetic resonance imaging (MRI) machines. The Pavilion also became home to the center's new medical library, with its 15,000 volumes and 340 medical and professional journals.[55]

Following Peterson to the podium at the dedication ceremony for the Francis Scott Key Pavilion was James Block, who succeeded Heyssel as president of The Johns Hopkins Hospital and Health System in 1992 and who, Peterson noted, had followed Heyssel's example by allowing him free rein "to continue the course that had been set" at what henceforth was to be known as the Johns Hopkins Bayview Medical Center. Block praised both his predecessor and Peterson for the astonishing accomplishments on Eastern Avenue and put them into national perspective:

"While other cities are struggling with their city hospitals; while city hospitals throughout the United States, in many cases, are finding it extremely difficult to provide quality care—or to sustain care at all—to those in need of the services of city hospitals, we have here, as a result of the vision of Robert Heyssel, the greatest conversion of a city hospital that exists in this country," Block said. The Pavilion also reflected the image "of the man who made it happen, Ron Peterson," he added.[56]

Michael Johns, dean of the Hopkins School of Medicine, also recognized the remarkable position that the Bayview Medical Center had come to occupy in the course of its unprecedented revitalization.

"This really... is a unique location, because it's one of the few places where city, state and federal programs come together with university and Johns Hopkins Health System programs—all on one campus," Johns noted. "I don't know that there's any other place where this really comes together in the same way."[57]

Peterson had invited former mayor, now Governor William Donald Schaefer to be the keynote speaker at the dedication. Schaefer, beaming at all that had taken place at the once-beleaguered City Hospitals in the past decade, proclaimed that "the smartest thing that we did in the city... [10 years ago] was to turn over the hospital to Johns Hopkins."

"Just look at what has been accomplished—the buildings, all... the great things that have happened here. It was a wonderful, wonderful smart move on the part of the city, and a great move on behalf of Hopkins."[58]

Within a year after FSK was renamed the Johns Hopkins Bayview Medical Center, Chesapeake Physicians, P.A., the pioneering faculty practice group whose collaboration with the Peterson team had been so crucial to Bayview's success, decided that it, too, should reflect its members' affiliation with the Johns Hopkins School of Medicine in its name. In 1995, the CPPA became Johns Hopkins Bayview Physicians, P.A. With 175 full-time and 130 part-time physicians, as well as more than 140 full- and part-time employees, it remained the core of the medical center's clinical activities.[59]

Changes and added responsibilities also were in store for several Bayview campus leaders. In May 1995, Block appointed Peterson the executive vice president and chief operating officer of the Johns Hopkins Health System. The executive vice presidency of the health system was a new position, "designed to bring a strong dimension of coordination and cohesion to our operations and strategic planning," Block explained in announcing the appointment.[60]

"For the first time, a principal officer of the Health System will have increased authority and resources to consolidate and blend support and administrative services across affiliate lines, and look for ways to work for the good of the greater whole," Block said.[61]

Even as he took on this new assignment, Peterson retained the presidency of Bayview, which he considered a model for what he hoped to do for the entire Hopkins health system. "This is an exciting opportunity for me to influence the development of an integrated delivery system at such an important juncture in the future of American health care," he wrote in a letter to his colleagues. "As part of my goals in this position, I have a strong commitment to build upon the progressive steps we have already taken here at Hopkins Bayview."[62]

The administrative leadership at Bayview also underwent some alteration. In early 1994, Bill Ward left Bayview to become a private consultant on finance and operations for health service organizations both nationally and internationally, working with such major institutions as the World Bank. He also became head of the M.H.S. degree program in health finance and management in Hopkins' School of Hygiene and Public Health, and taught finance in the School of Nursing's graduate business of nursing program and at the University of Maryland's School of Nursing.[63]

Ward's position as senior vice president for operations subsequently was filled by Gregory F. Schaffer, who initially was named vice present of support services at Bayview in August 1995. Schaffer, a native of Roxbury, Connecticut, earned his undergraduate degree from Central Connecticut State University and a master of science degree from Rensselaer Polytechnic Institute. A member of the American College of Healthcare Executives, the American Society for Hospital Engineering, and the American Society of Safety Engineers, Schaffer had been vice president for facilities and support services at Saint Vincent's Medical Center on Staten Island, New York, prior to joining the Bayview administration. He also held executive positions at the Hospital of Saint Raphael in New Haven, Connecticut, and McLean Hospital in Belmont, Massachusetts.[64]

Members of the Bayview faculty, like so many of their predecessors, were selected to assume top positions in national professional organizations. Maintaining the tradition of national leadership that long had been a hallmark of faculty members at Bayview, Andrew Munster of the Burn Center was elected president of the 3,000-member American Burn Association in August 1995; and Marvin M. Schuster, chief of the Division of Digestive Diseases, was chosen to become president-elect of the 5,600-member American College of Gastroenterology in November of that year.[65]

Bayview continued its steady increase in patient admissions, which was unmistakeable proof of the revitalized medical center's growing reputation for excellence. From 12,938 in 1990, admissions rose to 15,378 in 1995. By comparison, all the other Maryland hospitals saw their combined admissions plummet from 597,353 in 1990 to 553,891 in 1994, then recover to 570,301 in 1995—still 27,000 less than they had been at their peak five years earlier.[66]

Bayview's growth in admissions, coupled with the continuing rises in surgical procedures, clinic visits, emergency room visits and scrupulous attention to cost-effective operations, ensured that revenues remained on the black side of the ledger, averaging $3.25 million between 1990 and 1995.[67]

In retrospect, Peterson now thinks the renaming of the campus as the Johns Hopkins Bayview Medical Center and the opening of the stunningly modern Francis Scott Key Pavilion finally put to rest the Southeast Baltimore community's lingering concerns over the future of their long-troubled neighborhood hospital and Hopkins' ownership of it.

"That was the point at which, I believe, the community realized that we were going beyond the Baltimore City Hospitals era," Peterson notes. "They had always expressed concerns about the poor condition of the physical facilities, so I think the community at large was finally convinced that we were going beyond that."[68]

And far beyond that the Johns Hopkins Bayview Medical Center would continue to go.

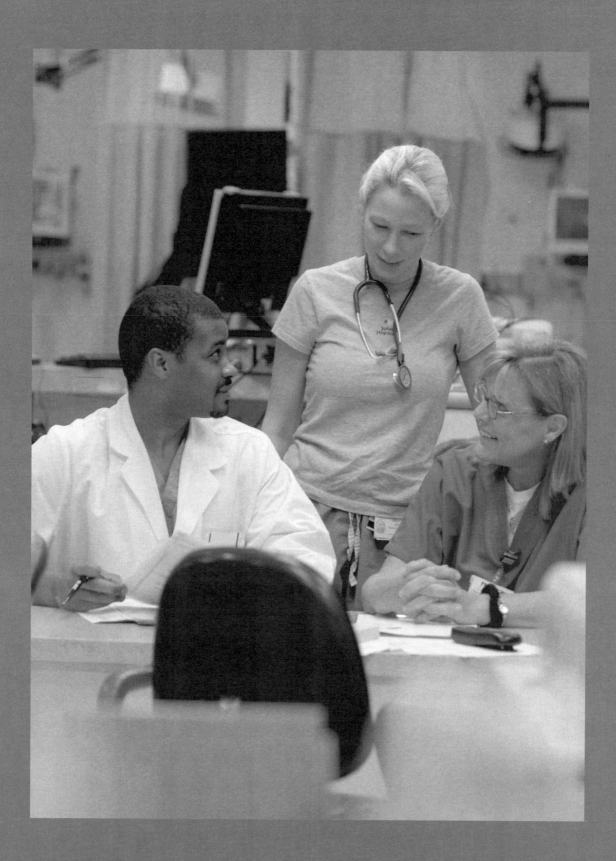

Sherwood Holloway, left, Kristen Nagel, standing, and Terry Littlejohn represent Hopkins Bayview's latest generation of caregivers. (Mike Ciesielski)

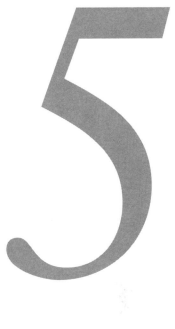

"Our true success is measured by the quality of people we have."

ADMINISTRATIVE TURMOIL HAD BEEN THE LEITMOTIF AT CITY Hospitals prior to its absorption by The Johns Hopkins Hospital in 1984. A dozen years later, the situation had been reversed. Major administrative alterations at Hopkins would lead, in turn, to leadership changes at the Hopkins Bayview Medical Center; some of the wizards who wrought wonders on Eastern Avenue went back to North Broadway to work their magic there. A changing of the guard during the second half of the 1990s prepared both institutions to enter the 21st century with renewed vigor.

When Hopkins Hospital's president, James Block, had asked Ron Peterson to fill the newly created position of executive vice president and chief operating officer of the Johns Hopkins Health System in May 1995, it was to solve problems of health system coordination that had eluded solution under Gennaro J. Vasile, a former chief operating officer of The Johns Hopkins Hospital, who had resigned that April.[1] Although Peterson remained president of Bayview, *The Sun* reported "the privately expressed opinion of many Hopkins employees that Mr. Peterson would be an ideal leader of the health system." Peterson told the paper he doubted that he, a non-physician, would be in a position to succeed a medical doctor such as Block, noting "a rich tradition of having physician leadership at the head of these medical institutions."[2] At the time, it seemed unlikely; a surprisingly short time later, it appeared inevitable.

The Johns Hopkins Hospital and The Johns Hopkins University School of Medicine had been separate entities since the university's founding a century earlier. They had collaborated brilliantly (albeit not without occasional

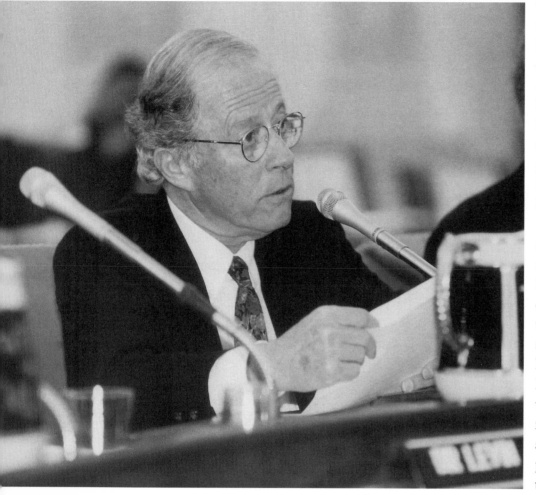

Marvin Schuster, retired chief of digestive diseases at Hopkins Bayview, is an international leader in the field. The Marvin M. Schuster Center for Gastrointestinal Motility and Digestive Disorders, opened in 1996, was the nation's first comprehensive research and care facility for people with gastrointestinal and motility disorders. Schuster, a former president of the American College of Gastroenterology, pioneered nonsurgical procedures for motility disorders and made significant discoveries about digestive diseases. (HBBMS)

tension) for decades. As medical historian John A. Kastor noted in his 2003 book, *Governance of Teaching Hospitals: Turmoil at Penn and Hopkins,* the comity between Hopkins Hospital and the school of medicine began eroding significantly in the early 1990s, when philosophical and personality conflicts arose between Block and the medical school dean, Michael Johns.[3]

In December 1995, Johns resigned as dean of the School of Medicine, announcing that he would move to Emory University by July 1, 1996.[4] A committee made of up members of the boards of trustees for the university, Hopkins Hospital and Johns Hopkins Medicine decided that revolutionary change was needed in the way the hospital and the school of medicine were run. With astonishing alacrity, the committee completed a plan by February 1996 to consolidate the leadership of Hopkins Medicine, putting the hospital and the school of medicine under the control of a single leader for the first time.

The new leader would serve both as dean of the School of Medicine and as chief executive officer of the hospital, or the "dean/CEO" of the medical enterprise. With Michael Johns scheduled to leave the deanship by July, Daniel Nathans, a Nobel Prize-winning scientist who was then the university's interim president, asked Edward D. Miller, director of the Department of Anesthesiology, to take over as interim dean in February 1996.[5]

Evidently unhappy with the pending reorganization of Hopkins Medicine, James Block resigned the hospital presidency in August 1996. Ron Peterson was chosen to become acting president of the hospital. The next month, William Brody, a former director of the Department of Radiology at Hopkins Hospital who had become provost of the University of Minnesota's medical center, returned to Hopkins as president of the university. The following December, the hospital trustees decided to remove the "acting" from Peterson's title and confirmed him as the hospital's tenth president, making him the first non-physician in half a century to run the institution.[6] With Peterson's support, Miller was selected to become the first dean/CEO of Hopkins Medicine in January 1997 (removing the "acting" from his title and giving him overall control of Hopkins Medicine as CEO). In February 1997, Peterson was named president of the Johns Hopkins Health System.[7]

When the administrative dust finally settled on North Broadway, The Johns Hopkins Hospital had a new leadership team of Edward Miller and Ron Peterson, who worked extremely well together. Bayview found itself sharing its president, Peterson, with its parent institution and the other entities in the Johns Hopkins Health System. Bayview also was

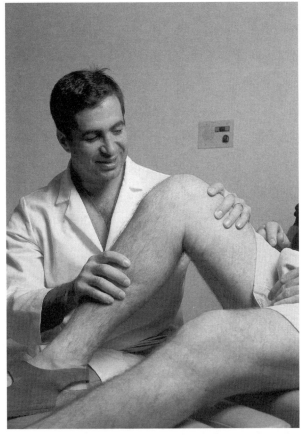

James Wenz (1964-2004) was a brilliant and innovative orthopedic surgeon and chairman of the Department of Orthopaedic Surgery at Hopkins Bayview at the time of his death in a tragic traffic accident in which his wife, child psychiatrist **Lidia Wenz**, also died. As an attending surgeon at Bayview and The Johns Hopkins Hospital, Wenz concentrated on total hip and total knee replacement surgery, the treatment of osteonecrosis, revision surgery for failed joint replacements and the use of cartilage in transplantation. Some of these advanced techniques incorporated minimally invasive procedures. He performed hundreds of hip replacements through a four-inch incision, rather than the standard 10- to 12-inch opening. Frank Frassica, chairman of the Department of Orthopaedic Surgery at Hopkins, says Wenz was "the most brilliant innovator and technical surgeon ever to graduate from the Johns Hopkins orthopedic surgery residency program." (HBBMS)

sharing its executive vice president with Hopkins Hospital. When he had become acting president of Hopkins Hospital in mid-1996, Peterson had asked Judy Reitz to join him on North Broadway as senior vice president for operations of the hospital, but she also retained her position at Bayview, just as he had. Peterson says he chose to retain the presidency of Bayview at that time because "there was not an heir apparent, and I decided to hold on to the position while deciding both the nature of the future reporting relationship to me, as well as the qualities I would need in a successor."[8]

Sharing its leadership with Hopkins Hospital did not in any way diminish the momentum of medical and physical plant advances at Bayview in the 1990s, with new buildings and innovative new clinical programs arising on Eastern Avenue as they had for the preceding decade.

In May 1996, ground was broken for a new ambulatory care center to replace the existing outpatient department's dispersed and outdated offices with a centralized, convenient location. The $13 million, three-story, 98,900-square-foot Bayview Medical Offices, completed in 1999, connected to the acute care hospital and housed such primary care services as general internal medicine, gynecology, obstetrics and pediatrics. Each medical specialty was given a separate reception room, waiting area and spacious exam rooms. To help children feel comfortable, the pediatrics rooms included a play area and exam tables that looked like animals. Specialty services in the new center

Gregory Schaffer succeeded Ronald Peterson as president of the Johns Hopkins Bayview Medical Center in 1999. His late father, Fred Schaffer, a student in Baltimore before becoming a dairy farmer in Connecticut, remembered the old City Hospitals from the 1930s. Though the elder Mr. Schaffer could not recognize much of the modern campus on a return visit, he instantly remembered the familiar entrance to the old acute care hospital, seen behind Schaffer, that now faces the campus's rose garden. (Keith Weller)

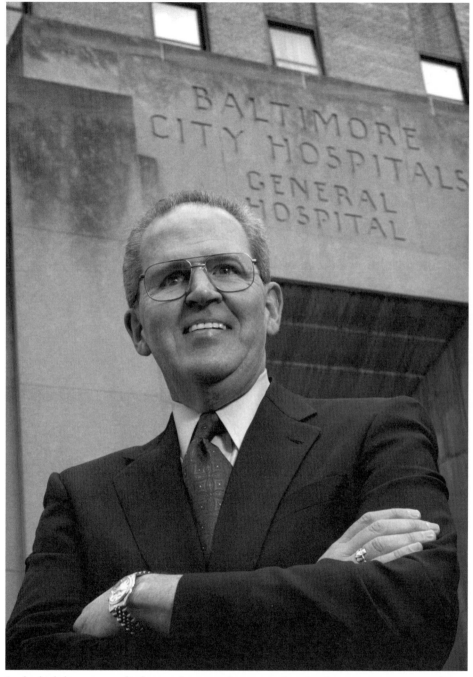

included burn, cardiology, dermatology, endocrinology, gastroenterology, hematology/oncology, imaging services (including X-ray, mammography and ultrasound), minor surgery, neurodiagnostic lab, neurology, ophthalmology, orthopedics, otolaryngology (ear, nose and throat), plastic surgery, podiatry, urology and vascular lab.[9]

Continuing its tradition as a focal point of medical innovation, in November 1996 Bayview opened the Marvin M. Schuster Center for Gastrointestinal Motility and Digestive Disorders, the nation's first comprehensive research and care facility for people with these conditions. Named for the chief of digestive diseases at Bayview and an international leader in the field, the 10,000 square-foot Schuster Center featured a fully equipped endoscopy suite consisting of four procedure rooms, an eight-bed recovery room and a separate waiting room for endoscopy patients.[10]

Schuster, then president of the American College of Gastroenterology, had many firsts in his field. He was the first director of a gastrointestinal division trained both in medicine and psychiatry; the first to form a gastrointestinal division with completely integrated full-time psychology and medical faculty; and the first to establish a gastrointestinal pain management center within a gastrointestinal division. A member of the Johns Hopkins faculty since 1961, he also pioneered nonsurgical procedures for some motility disorders and made significant discoveries about such digestive diseases as irritable bowel syndrome (IBS), which afflicts nearly 15 percent of the nation's population; gastro-esophageal reflux disease (GERD), which causes frequent heartburn and difficulty in swallowing, among other symptoms; fecal incontinence; and chronic intestinal pseudo-obstruction (CIP), which afflicts more than 50,000 people.[11]

Under Schuster's leadership, an interdisciplinary team of physicians and scientists at the new center began exploring the causes of and developing effective new treatments for motility disorders, which affect some 35 million Americans and can result in severe abdominal pain, nausea, vomiting, maldigestion, weight loss, diarrhea, constipation and incontinence.[12] Within five months, the importance of the work at the Schuster Center prompted the Jacob and Hilda Blaustein Foundation in Baltimore to pledge $200,000 to fund patient research there.[13]

The Blaustein Foundation was just one of many local supporters of initiatives at Bayview. Contributions from area residents and the business community helped boost the hospital's capital campaign, launched in 1992, to $3.2 million, just $300,000 short of its $3.5 million goal, by 1995. The money was targeted for renovating the older campus buildings and for aiding its trauma center, emergency department, imaging center, burn unit and geriatrics center.[14] In December 1996, the Baltimore Ravens football team created the Baltimore Ravens-Hopkins Bayview Kids Fund to help pediatric patients. A year later, the Ravens Wives Association joined with the Metropolitan Fire Fighters to host the first Baltimore Ravens FANtastic Charity Event in December 1997. Modeled after a football game—complete with a tailgate party, pregame and postgame shows, photo and autograph sessions with Ravens players and a silent auction of sports memorabilia—the gala raised $109,000 to establish a pediatric burn center at Bayview.[15]

The community had reason to be proud of its hospital. Its staff regularly was responsible for important medical discoveries and technical breakthroughs, and the hospital itself undertook continuous efforts to provide services its community needed, both on campus and in the neighborhoods.

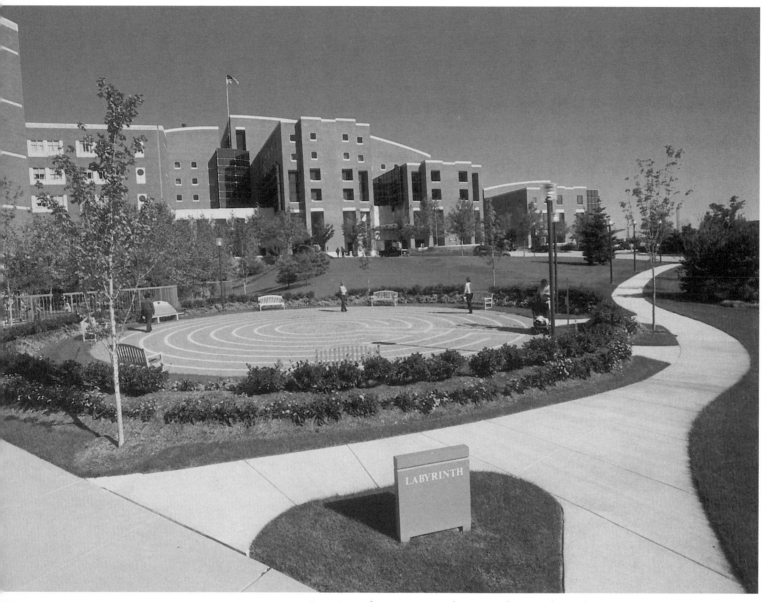

Labyrinths have symbolized hope, healing and spirit for thousands of years. The Hopkins Bayview labyrinth, the first on the East Coast placed in a health care setting, was funded by the TKF Foundation and opened in June 2000. It has become a popular spot for relaxation, reflection and recreation. (HBBMS)

Bayview physicians revolutionized procedures for operating on living kidney donors, pioneered minimally invasive hip surgery and other surgical breakthroughs, and conducted landmark research on the causes of obesity.[16]

Lloyd E. Ratner, chief of transplantation at Bayview, and Louis Kavoussi, chief of urology, performed what was believed to be the first surgical procedure of its kind in November 1995. Using a laparoscope and minimal incisions, they operated simultaneously on a living kidney donor, a 25-year-old man, and on his mother, the recipient of the kidney. Kavoussi, wielding a robotic arm to control the laparoscope (a small lighted telescope), inserted it into a half-inch incision in the donor's body. The laparoscope enabled Kavoussi and Ratner to view and then remove the donor's kidney. When the organ was nearly removed, Ratner went into an adjoining operating room, prepared the recipient for her kidney transplant, and performed it. The donor was out of the hospital in just two days, on his way to recovery; the recipient recovered swiftly, too.[17]

"In past surgeries, incisions had to be made halfway around the donor's flank," and the donor spent nearly six days in the hospital and required up to three months for total recuperation, Ratner told *Bayview News.* Laparoscopic live-donor nephrectomies meant donors would spend less time in the hospital with reduced scarring, less postoperative pain, and speedier recoveries. All these improvements, Ratner and Kavoussi hoped, would encourage a major increase in the number of kidney donations.

Minimally invasive surgery techniques were also being pioneered in Bayview's orthopedics department, where James Wenz became one of the first physicians in the country to use a "mini hip" procedure, totally replacing a patient's hip through a four-inch incision. Traditional total hip replacement surgery involves an incision approximately 10 to 12 inches long and frequently causes significant trauma to leg muscles. The minimally invasive technique perfected by Wenz doesn't affect the abductor muscles in the leg, resulting in less pain and quicker recovery for patients. Prior to Wenz's tragic death in January 2004, when he and his wife, Lidia Wenz, a child psychiatrist, were killed in an auto accident, he had performed hundreds of the minimally invasive total hip replacements and won international acclaim for his surgical skills.[18]

Bayview's orthopedic services became even more comprehensive. A new trauma clinic was established to immediately handle patients arriving in the ER with fractures and sprains. A specialized team was created to deal with hip fractures, alternative (nonsurgical) treatment for arthritis and joint reconstruction. A new spine service was headed by John Carbone; treatment of hand-related problems was overseen by Peter Innis; shoulder, elbow and hand injuries were treated by William Beatie; foot and ankle surgery was offered under the supervision of Ronald Byank; pediatric orthopedics was headed by Michael Ain. Bayview even offered a sports medicine program geared to older active adults—those weekend warriors who discovered during exercise or sports that they weren't as young as they used to be.[19]

The Department of Surgery at Bayview boomed during the 1990s. Between 1993 and 1998, the number of its operating rooms nearly doubled and surgery figures soared, reaching 625 surgeries in January 1998 alone, an all-time monthly high. "The numbers don't tell the real story," John Harmon, chairman of the surgery department, told *Bayview News.* "Our true success is measured by the quality of people we have." Not only were the surgeons superbly qualified, but the anesthesia and nursing staffs in surgery managed the burgeoning caseloads with panache, Harmon said. He and Jeffrey Bender, Mark Duncan and Thomas Magnuson provided extraordinary expertise in

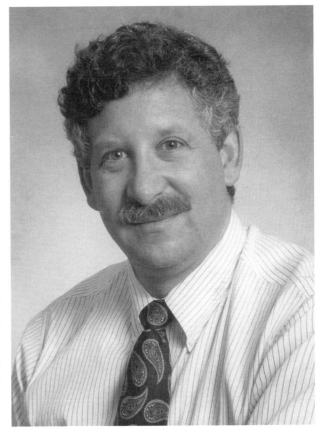

L. Reuven Pasternak, the last president of Hopkins Bayview Physicians before its merger with the School of Medicine's Clinical Practice Association (CPA), was chosen by Dean Edward Miller to be the first vice dean for the Bayview campus. Pasternak had years of experience as chief of anesthesiology and associate dean for clinical affairs at Bayview and, before that, as first division chief for ambulatory anesthesiology at Hopkins Hospital. After the integration of the faculty practice groups, he became chairman of the CPA's operations oversight committee. (HBBMS)

gastrointestinal and endocrine surgical procedures such as laparoscopic gall-bladder surgery, esophageal reflux laparoscopic surgery, gastric bypass surgery, colon surgery, gastroesophageal surgery, pancreatic surgery, thyroid surgery, and parathyroid surgery.[20]

The operating rooms at Bayview were not the only venues producing impressive results; so were the laboratories. In 1986, Alan Shuldiner, Kristi Silver and Jeremy Walston, collaborating with colleagues in Sweden, Finland and France, reported in the *New England Journal of Medicine* that they had discovered a genetic flaw that made certain people more susceptible to obesity and to the onset of type 2 diabetes. They found that a defect in a gene that makes a protein called the beta-3-adrenergic receptor, which helps regulate metabolism and fat breakdown in abdominal fat cells, causes individuals with the faulty gene to burn fewer calories and store fat more easily, especially around their middles. Such spare tires, or pot bellies, can signal an increased risk of heart attack or type 2 diabetes, which can lead to significant problems including blindness, strokes, kidney disease, circulatory problems and heart disease.[21]

The most exciting aspect of the discovery by Shuldiner, Silver and Walston was its potential for suggesting new ways to treat both obesity and type 2 diabetes. New medications aimed at altering a person's metabolism by selectively targeting the beta-3 receptor could be developed to treat the problems prompted by the defective gene. Even a simple blood test—

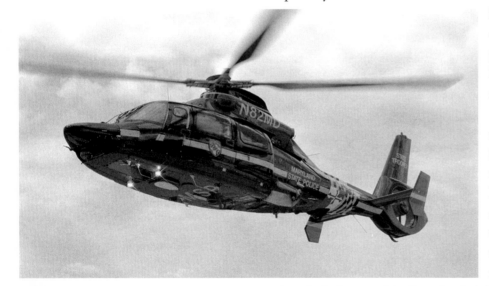

Maryland State Police Medevac helicopters rush critically injured patients, most of them suffering from burns, to Hopkins Bayview. In fiscal year 2004, of the Bayview Regional Burn Center's 313 admissions, 51 were patients arriving via state police helicopters. (Courtesy Richard Yienger, Maryland State Police.)

already being used in Bayview's labs—could identify people who have the genetic defect, perhaps in childhood. That would be the best time for them to begin lifestyle practices of regular exercise and a healthier diet to prevent obesity, despite their inherited predilection to put on pounds. "If you control your diet and exercise often, in most cases you can override the effects of this genetic burden," Shuldiner told *Bayview News*.[22]

A growing interest in the health prognoses of its Southeast Baltimore neighbors led Bayview to join with several other regional hospitals in launching the year-long Community Health Assessment Project (CHAP) in 1996. Seeking to identify health risk factors and specific unmet community needs, Bayview enlisted the help of community leaders to assist in coordinating the compilation of data from household surveys, focus groups, physician questionnaires and census results. After surveying nearly 800 area residents, the investigators painted a sobering picture of Bayview's prospective patients: a group that was heavier, smoked more and drank more than the average resident of the

Baltimore metropolitan area, and that also was aging rapidly. More than 40 percent of the survey respondents were overweight, and heart disease was the number one killer in the community.[23]

The CHAP results "have tremendous implications for the way we treat patients, the way we train health care providers and how we develop new community health programs," Gayle Adams, Bayview's long-time director of community relations, told *Bayview News*, the publication the hospital distributed throughout its region. Bayview found the survey so helpful that it plans to conduct another comprehensive one, beginning in 2004.[24]

Bayview ratcheted up efforts to reach community residents earlier than ever to improve their health. It launched the Bayview maternity care campaign in July 1997, offering expanded educational materials and classes devoted to childbirth preparation, parenting and baby safety. It even included classes for children—the future big brothers and big sisters of the babies yet to be born.[25]

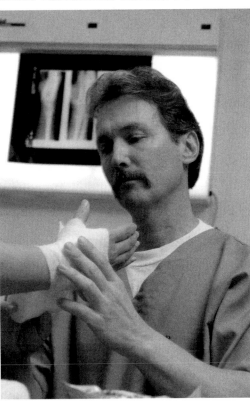

The **helping hands** of orthotist **Rob Rawson** begin preparations for a cast in the Hopkins Bayview orthopedics department. **(HBBMS)**

Initiatives were undertaken to ensure that quality health care would be just around the corner for Bayview's community members—or even at their fingertips. In 1997, Bayview launched its Web site, http://www.jhbmc.jhu.edu, providing descriptions and phone numbers of all of the hospital's major services, together with health advice and other useful information, including back issues of *Bayview News*.[26] Johns Hopkins Bayview Physicians, P.A., added health centers in Dundalk and the Harford County corridor. The group opened an 8,000-square-foot facility in the Merritt Park Shopping Center in August 1998, providing internal medicine, pediatrics, mammography and radiology, as well as concentrating the physical therapy services there that previously had been offered in Dundalk Village and Harbor View. The group's successful Riverside center in Harford County was expanded by 3,000 square feet to accommodate more patients.[27] By 1999, Bayview operated seven community clinics.[28]

The variety of educational programs and support groups offered at the medical center also grew. The outpatient pulmonary rehabilitation program held monthly meetings for patients with respiratory diseases. Blood pressure

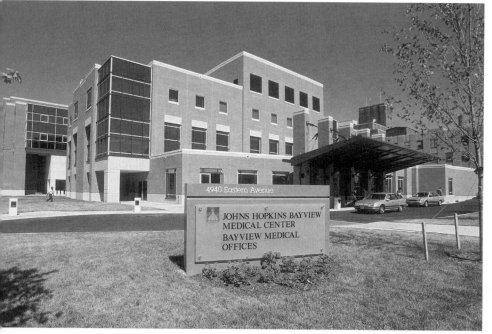

The Bayview Medical Offices, a $13 million, 98,900-square-foot building completed in 1999, houses the primary care services of general internal medicine, gynecology, obstetrics and pediatrics. Each service has a separate reception room, waiting area and spacious exam rooms. The pediatrics room features a play area and exam tables that look like animals. Among many specialty services in the center are burn, cardiology, dermatology, endocrinology, gastroenterology and imaging, including X-ray. (HBBMS)

screenings were offered monthly at the Eastpoint Mall food court. CPR techniques for treating adults, children and infants, pioneered at Bayview, were taught for a minimal fee. Cholesterol screenings were available at modest cost. Heart health displays, information and classes were offered. Support groups served breast cancer patients, burn survivors and their families, head and neck cancer patients, gastric surgery candidates, caregivers for frail elderly people, and the families of people addicted to drugs or alcohol.[29]

Given the growing number of elderly residents in its neighborhoods and its long history as an innovative site for senior care, Bayview was a natural fit for a new federal initiative, the Program of All-Inclusive Care for the Elderly (PACE). A national demonstration project of the Health Care Financing Administration (HCFA) funded by both Medicare and Medicaid, PACE was intended to help frail elderly people continue to live independently in their own communities and avoid premature admission to nursing homes. When it became one of only 15 health care facilities in the nation and the only one in Maryland to participate in PACE, Bayview created Hopkins ElderPlus in 1996 to provide acute and long-term care for seniors who required a nursing home level of care but could be treated in their neighborhoods with the help of a multidisciplinary health care team from the hospital.[30]

Hopkins ElderPlus provides preventive, rehabilitative, curative and support services, comprehensive prescription coverage and transportation to doctors' appointments and to the ElderPlus day care program. The average age of PACE enrollees is 80 and all have significant health problems, but Hopkins ElderPlus' preventive care efforts, like those of its counterparts elsewhere in the nation, effectively enable some 94 percent of the program's participants to stay out of long-term care facilities.[31]

Recognizing the barriers to obtaining health care, especially in the poorer neighborhoods of its community, Bayview took its services on the road. It purchased a $125,000 "Care-A-Van" in 1999 with a grant from the March of Dimes and contributions from the Kiwanis Club of East Baltimore (a longtime supporter of the Burn Center), the Bank of America, the Merrick Foundation, the Chesapeake Health Plan Foundation, and WBAL-AM Radio's "Kids Campaign." The 39-foot mobile clinic was outfitted with a consultation area, two exam rooms and a television for showing health-teaching videos. Focusing its efforts on preventive medicine and maternal and child health, the van traveled four days a week to medically underserved schools and community centers in Dundalk and Highlandtown. "We want to extend the hospital's doors," Michael Crocetti, chairman of Bayview's pediatrics department and medical director of the Care-A-Van, told *Bayview News*, "but we don't want to become a medical home." The goal of the van "is to connect people with services they need," such as nearby primary care, family services or the federal Women, Infants and Children (WIC) nutrition program.[32]

In the hospital itself, new services were begun and existing services enhanced. Bayview opened a five-bed neuroscience critical care unit (NSCCU) in 1997 for the expert staff specializing in diagnosis and treatment of patients with strokes, brain tumors, aneurysms, head injuries and other severe neurological disorders. It was one of the few centers in the country able to administer the only drug then approved to treat acute strokes—tissue plasminogen activator (tPA), a clot-busting drug newly approved by the U.S. Food and Drug Administration. Under co-directors Alessandro Olivi and Christopher J. Earley, the NSCCU expanded the range of Bayview's already exceptional neurosciences program, treating everything from sleep disorders to dementia, epilepsy, neuromuscular disease, neuropsychology, movement disorders, neuropsychology and neurovascular disease.[33]

Reaching far beyond its immediate neighborhood—which had many residents of Greek, Italian or Polish descent with strong ties to their homelands—Bayview launched a new international services program to provide consultation and care to patients from around the globe. "We want these people to know that we're here to meet their medical needs, as well as those of loved ones overseas," nurse Virginia C. Alinsao, director of international services marketing, told *Bayview News*. The international services staff was trained to help foreign patients and their families obtain visas, meet immigration requirements, find places to stay, arrange for translators during their visit, and help Bayview doctors maintain contact with the patient's medical

The **Care-A-Van,** a $125,000, 39-foot mobile clinic, began making its rounds in 1999, extending Hopkins Bayview's services to medically underserved schools and community centers. (HBBMS)

provider back home. The new program also offered a one-day, extensive "executive outpatient physical" for business travelers and people who were visiting family or friends in the United States. It also arranged with shipping companies to provide examinations, tests and treatment for sick sailors aboard foreign vessels docking in the Port of Baltimore.[34]

In Bayview's emergency department, one of the few centers in Maryland specially designed and staffed to deal with hazardous materials exposures—the Hazmat Referral Center—was created. It featured a special decontamination room equipped with showers designed to capture

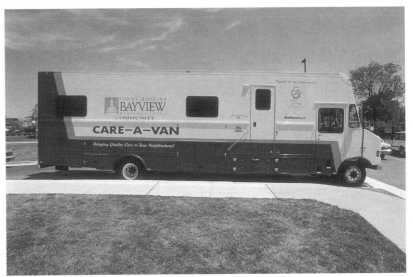

potentially hazardous runoff; and a specially trained emergency department hazmat team of physicians and nurses. Its location at Bayview was deemed especially appropriate because of the hospital's designation as an areawide trauma center and regional burn center. Initially established primarily to treat workers from local industries, where the potential for chemical-related accidents was high, the Hazmat Referral Center became an even more crucial component of Bayview's services after biochemical terrorism concerns arose following the September 11, 2001, terrorist attacks in New York and Washington, D.C.[35]

In the Regional Burn Center, a $75,000 gift from the Baltimore Metropolitan Fire Fighters and the Burn Center Community Fund enabled Bayview to purchase a laser scanner that could be used to produce a therapeutic facial mask. Use of the mask reduces facial scarring during burn treatment and recovery; Bayview's is the first burn center in the country to offer state-of-the-art total contact burn masks. With the new equipment, the entire scanning process is completed in as little as eight seconds—a dramatic improvement from traditional mask-making, which can take up to two hours. The new method is neither frightening nor painful, so it is far more patient-friendly. Since Bayview began using the laser scanner to create burn masks, other burn centers have adopted the same technology.[36]

The excellence of Bayview's physicians continued to be recognized and celebrated by peers and patients. In 1997 alone, five of the hospital's staff members were cited for their exceptional accomplishments. John R. Burton, director of geriatric medicine, received the Physician of the Year award from the National Association for Home Care, honoring his commitment to serving the needs of the frail elderly and to conducting research and education that emphasized the importance of helping seniors live independently. Andrew Munster and Robert Spence, co-directors of the Baltimore Regional Burn Center, were named by *Baltimore* magazine as the best in the area for burn/surgery treatment. Sharon Walsh of the Behavioral Pharmacology Research Unit received the Presidential Early Career Award for Scientists and Engineers at the White House in recognition of her development of a model for cocaine withdrawal that may lead to the discovery of new treatments for cocaine abuse. Jimmy B. Zachary of the Division of Renal Medicine was honored by the National Kidney Foundation for his lifetime of work dedicated to caring for patients with kidney disease. As founder of the Division of Renal Medicine at Bayview in 1974, when it still was City Hospitals, Zachary was one of the first physicians to perform hemodialysis treatments in the city. He also organized the team that performed the first kidney transplant in Baltimore.[37]

As the 1990s came to a close, the changing of the guard in Hopkins Medicine that had begun in mid-decade reached the Bayview campus with the appointment of a new leadership team. In August 1999, Ron Peterson relinquished the presidency of Bayview and joined with the Bayview board of trustees in appointing Gregory Schaffer as his successor. Elizabeth B. Concordia, Bayview's vice president of clinical services, was appointed executive vice president and chief operating officer, succeeding Judy Reitz.[38] (Concordia later became president of several hospitals belonging to the University of Pittsburgh Medical Center, and senior vice president of its academic and community hospitals division.)

Another leadership change occurred that summer, when Chester Schmidt, one of the founders of Hopkins Bayview Physicians and its president for more than 20 years, handed over the presidency of the physicians' practice group to Reuven Pasternak, a former chairman of the Department of Anesthesiology and of the medical board at Bayview. Pasternak, a second-generation graduate of The Johns Hopkins University, also was vice chairman for health system affairs, the Department of Anesthesiology and Critical Care Medicine at the Johns Hopkins School of Medicine and the Johns Hopkins Health System. Schmidt accepted the newly created post of Bayview Physicians' medical director and continued as chairman of the Department of Psychiatry at the medical center.[39]

As the old century wound down, Hopkins Bayview's numbers kept going up. Other hospitals in Maryland experienced relatively flat growth in outpatient services, but Bayview's outpatient figures rose an astonishing 4 percent to 5 percent annually. Its admissions soared from 13,000 per year in 1995 to 20,000 by 2000. When Hopkins acquired it in 1984, the old City Hospitals had ranked a poor fourth in overall outpatient and admissions figures in its primary service area, behind Franklin Square, Hopkins and Church Home and Hospital (which ultimately would be closed). By 2000, Bayview had climbed to number one, ahead of Franklin Square and Hopkins Hospital.[40]

Entering its third century, Bayview's prospects were bright.

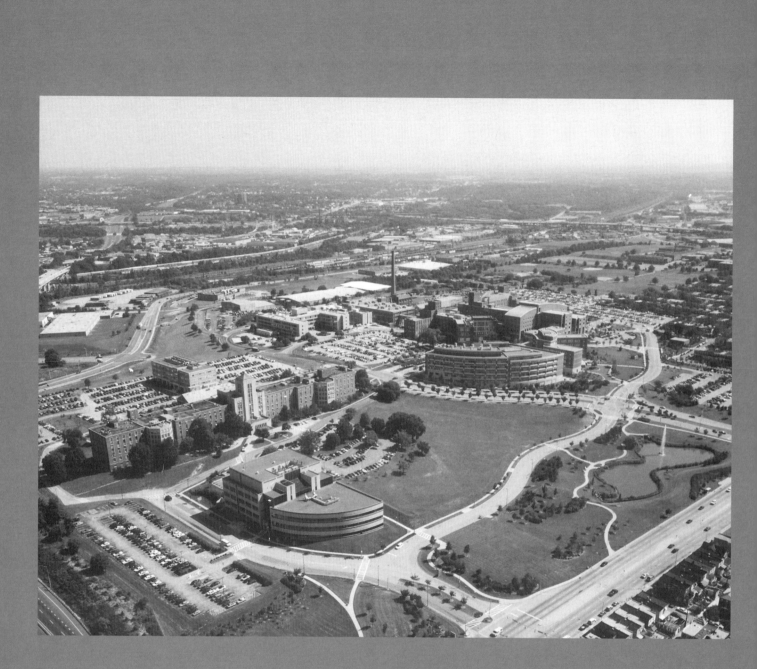

An aerial view of Bayview in 2000.

"What will Bayview do for an encore?"

AS THE YEAR 2000 APPROACHED, JOHNS HOPKINS BAYVIEW MEDICAL Center planned for what *Bayview News* ominously described as "the greatest potential computer glitch of all time," the ballyhooed Y2K information system breakdown.[1]

Stemming from the common computer programming practice of using only the last two digits to designate a calendar year, the Y2K problem, postulated by experts around the world, was that computers might not recognize or respond correctly when 1999 rolled over to 2000. Would Bayview's computers think it was 1900 again, back when the hospital was called Bay View Asylum?

Robert S. Ross, senior director of support services at Hopkins Bayview, led a team of experts from the facilities engineering, clinical engineering and information services offices that spent two years preparing for the worst scenario, figuring that a complete computer malfunction could affect everything from X-ray equipment and EKG machines to ventilators and elevators. The Hopkins Bayview team coordinated its efforts with those of the Johns Hopkins Health System as well as with Baltimore City, Bell Atlantic, Baltimore Gas and Electric Company and emergency service providers.[2]

January 1, 2000, arrived. Nothing happened.

Along with the sigh of relief and many bemused chuckles came the knowledge that Hopkins Bayview had been prepared for any disaster, as a top-tier hospital is supposed to be.

The computer gurus' concerted efforts were not the only evidence of

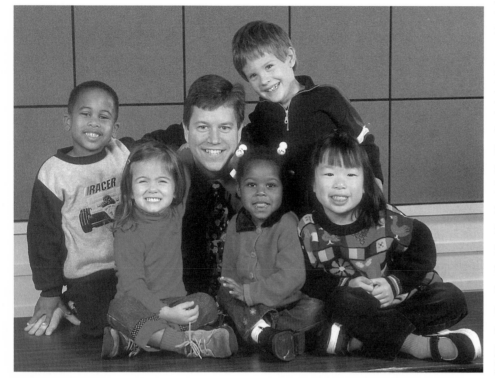

Michael Crocetti, chief of pediatrics at Hopkins Bayview, stresses the different requirements of patients in the Children's Medical Practice. "Children aren't just smaller versions of adults," he says. "They have different medical problems and special psychological and social needs." The Children's Medical Practice emphasizes preventive health maintenance and offers a private practice model of care in a hospital setting. (HBBMS)

Bayview's significant preparations for real or imagined emergencies. In 1998, Bayview had been designated a Level II adult trauma center by the Maryland Institute for Emergency Medical Services Systems (MIEMSS), one of only five such centers in the state.[3] In addition to being the only state-designated regional burn center, Bayview exceeded the state's requirements for its trauma center designation. It offered the required round-the-clock emergency department, intensive care units and operating rooms; a constantly available trauma surgeon and anesthesiologist; on-call orthopedic and neurosurgeons and a physician in the intensive care unit 24 hours a day. It also had enhanced support in orthopedics and neurology, as well as surgical residency coverage 24 hours a day, seven days a week.[4]

Demands on Hopkins Bayview's emergency department, even in normal times, were increasing enormously. In 2000, nearly 50,000 people visited the ED, a 29 percent rise in visits since 1994. It was estimated the number might increase another 47 percent by 2005. The waiting area was renovated and the triage area expanded so staff could see patients more quickly.[5]

The changing of the guard that began late in the 1990s continued with the decision by nationally renowned rheumatologist David Hellmann, executive vice chairman and residency program director for the Department of Medicine at The Johns Hopkins Hospital, to move over to Hopkins Bayview in 2000 to chair its department of medicine, succeeding Philip Zieve.[6]

Hellmann's move from Broadway to Eastern Avenue had special significance for many at Bayview, who still felt a lingering sense of historical condescension from their colleagues at Hopkins Hospital. (For years, a popular T-shirt sold at the Hopkins gift shop read: "It's Hard to Be Humble When You're from Johns Hopkins."[7]) Trustee Robert D.H. Harvey, a member of the board of both institutions, says that the Bayview board strove to "break down the kind of barrier that existed between Hopkins and the old City Hospitals."[8]

"City Hospitals was thought of as sort of second-class, and Hopkins didn't want to say that City Hospitals was a brother and equal to it," Harvey remembers.

Burton D'Lugoff recalls that generations of Hopkins medical students had done considerable portions of their training at the old City Hospitals and continued to do so at Bayview, where the medical staff had appointments to the faculty of the Hopkins School of Medicine for decades. Yet, he says, there remained "a tremendous sense downtown [at Hopkins Hospital] that the moment you left the campus, all knowledge ceased; that it only occurred under the dome" of the landmark Hopkins administration building.[9] And Chester Schmidt notes that "living with an 800-pound gorilla," meaning Hopkins, "isn't always easy."[10]

Strained relationships between a parent institution and its subordinates are hardly unique to Hopkins and Bayview. "That is extant in every academic medical center," notes D'Lugoff. Thus, David Hellmann's decision to move east to Hopkins Bayview was regarded by many insiders as a major change in the dynamics between the two institutions.

"I can't tell you how important that was, because he came from across town," says Greg Schaffer. "He's a person of high stature, very well respected at the School of Medicine, at Hopkins Hospital, who transitioned over to Bayview and has committed himself to really growing the program here to be on a par with Hopkins Hospital.[11]

"When David came here, it caused a lot of people to take a second look at Bayview," Schaffer says. "If someone of his stature was coming here, there must be something good going on. As a result of that, he's recruited some excellent division directors within the Department of Medicine and others have followed him in other departments—quality, excellent people who could go anywhere else in the country if they wanted to."[12]

Changes in the leadership at the school of medicine also contributed to altering the atmosphere, as did the absorption in 2002 of Johns Hopkins Bayview Physicians by the Clinical Practice Association, the faculty practice group at Hopkins Hospital, Schaffer notes.

"Ed Miller has pretty much put an end to people looking down their noses at Bayview. Hopkins Hospital has a new chief of surgery, Julie Freischlag, who is as much involved here as she is there. And Harold Fox, chief of Ob/Gyn, is involved out here and over there. It's a very different situation than it was just six or seven years ago," concludes Schaffer.[13]

Because fewer of the physicians at Bayview received outside grants to provide a portion of their salaries (unlike many of the full-time faculty at Hopkins Hospital) and because many Bayview patients had their medical expenses covered by managed care companies that often paid less for services, the Johns Hopkins Bayview Physicians group was losing money by the early 2000s.[14] Despite revenues of $74 million in 2000-2001, Bayview Physicians recorded a $3 million loss that fiscal year. Modern physician practice plans require substantial administrative support to maintain their billing operations, and the Clinical Practice Association at Hopkins Hospital had the administrative

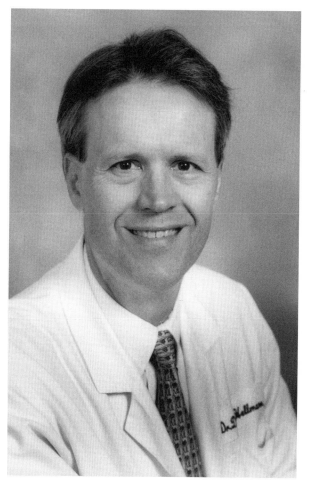

David Hellmann chose to move from Hopkins Hospital to Hopkins Bayview in 2000 to become the new chairman of the Department of Medicine. Hellmann, a renowned rheumatologist, has recruited exceptional division directors within the Department of Medicine, attracted highly regarded individuals to join Hopkins Bayview's other departments, and committed himself to developing programs at Bayview that equal those at Hopkins Hospital. **(HBBMS)**

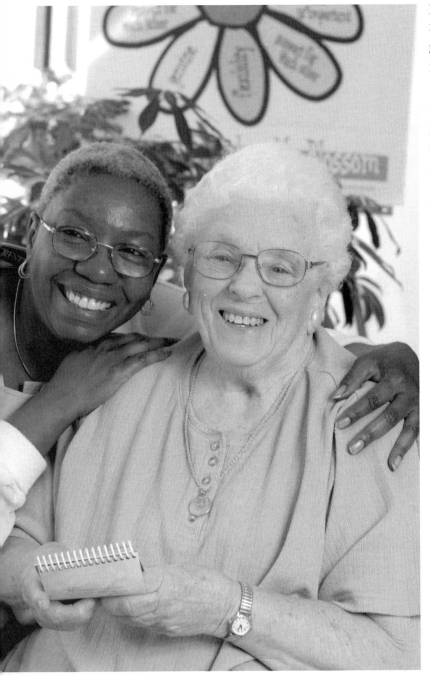

Warmth and caring are the hallmark of the Johns Hopkins Bayview Care Center, where registered nurse **Jessie Goins**, left, enjoys chatting with patient **Clara Budd.** (Mike Ciesielski)

power that Hopkins Medicine's leaders felt was needed at Bayview. A merger of the two practice groups was seen as the solution to Bayview Physicians' money woes.

Consolidation of the two practice groups under the CPA name created one of the largest academic group practices in the country. When the integration was completed in January 2002, Edward Miller said, "We needed to combine the strengths of the faculty practices at Bayview and East Baltimore to reflect one voice and work together to develop additional clinical centers of excellence and expand research and teaching opportunities on both campuses."[15] Emphasizing that the merger would not diminish Bayview physicians' dedication to treating patients in Bayview's community, Reuven Pasternak said, "Except for changes in the name on bills, the merger should be invisible to patients." The financial result of the merger was not invisible, however; it produced a half-million dollars in savings within a year, according to Pasternak.[16]

To coordinate the merger, Miller had created the new position of vice dean for the Bayview campus early in 2001, and he asked Pasternak to assume its duties. Pasternak had years of experience as both chief of anesthesiology and associate dean for clinical affairs at Bayview and, before that, as first division chief for ambulatory anesthesiology at Hopkins Hospital. He is, in Miller's words, "a quintessential Hopkins family man," with a father, a brother, a sister and cousins, holding more than 30 Hopkins degrees among them. (Pasternak's wife was a former associate director of pediatric nursing at Hopkins Hospital.) As the integration the faculty groups was worked out, Pasternak chaired an oversight committee of the Bayview clinical chiefs, served as chief advocate for the Bayview-based faculty, and was the main liaison between Bayview and representatives of the school of medicine's dean's office. After the faculty integration, he became chair of the Clinical Practice Association's operations oversight committee, along with his other duties.[17]

"The integration of the faculty practices has been a huge thing," says Schaffer. "It has better aligned the faculty to serve the needs of both institutions. Where there had been a sense that we were in competition with one another, that is gone. And the chairmen of the School of Medicine are responsible for the activities of the departments at both hospitals. They have a chief on site for Bayview, but they nevertheless ultimately are responsible for the department."[18]

Bayview departments continued to grow physically and programmatically and to win acclaim for their clinical and research achievements.

In the annual medical school rankings compiled by *U.S. News & World Report* magazine, Johns Hopkins' geriatrics program, based at Bayview, was named number one in its field of specialty programs in 2003. The outstanding care provided in Bayview's intensive care unit earned it recognition as one of the top 100 ICUs in the nation from the Solucient Leadership Institute, which collected data from 1,200 hospitals to conduct an independent study of ICU operations. As the birthplace 43 years earlier of the country's first ICU under Peter Safar, Bayview remained a beacon of superior treatment for patients requiring intensive attention.[19]

In addition to the emergency department expansion, the new Comprehensive Vascular Center (CVC) opened a streamlined clinic to provide a complete range of vascular services in one location, offering the latest in diagnostic and surgical facilities for treating atherosclerosis, peripheral vascular disease or poor circulation. Because treatment of vascular problems often brings several medical specialties into play, patients frequently were inconvenienced by having to make separate appointments at different locations. "Our new center brings the care team together in one clinic and makes the process easier for everyone," Rita Falcone, director of the CVC, told *Bayview News*.[20]

The Bayview Medical Offices was completed in 2001, when the last remaining floor was fitted out to provide new homes for several outpatient clinics in general internal medicine, ophthalmology, otolaryngology (ENT), audiology, and general surgery, plastic surgery and neurosurgery. These new offices made the "one-stop shopping" locale for outpatient health care needs, initially opened in 1999, even more convenient for Bayview patients.[21]

The physical rehabilitation department, long housed in an old part of the medical center, was given a new, centralized 11,500-square-foot location in the main hospital in 2002. Providing occupational therapy, physical therapy and speech language pathology services to nearly 500 new outpatients and 1,000 new inpatients a month, the renovated center enabled the rehabilitation department to serve its clients more efficiently with, among other features, separate gymnasiums for the inpatients and the outpatients. Bayview therapists in all the disciplines took part in designing the new space.[22]

The future of orthopedics arrived at Bayview when the new International Center for Orthopedic Advancement opened in 2002. The center, which has both a surgical suite and an instrument development laboratory with computer-controlled materials-testing equipment, is a place where surgeons collaborate with engineers to develop new orthopedic implants and surgical

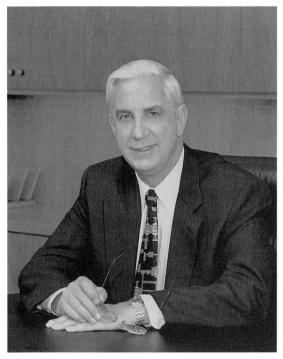

Edward D. Miller, the first chief executive officer of Johns Hopkins Medicine, 13th dean of The Johns Hopkins University School of Medicine and vice president for medicine of The Johns Hopkins University, has been a strong advocate of close collaboration between all entities of Johns Hopkins Medicine. (JHMOCC)

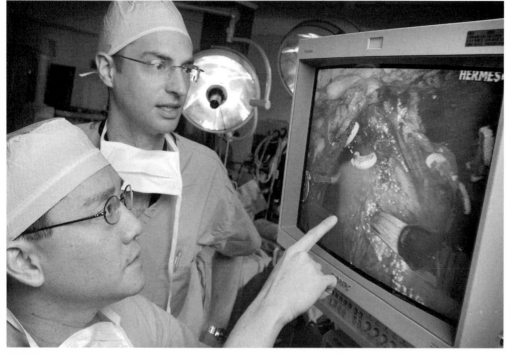

Urologists **Li-Ming Su** and **Christian Pavlovich** at Hopkins Bayview are experts in minimally invasive surgery for prostate cancer, one of the greatest health concerns for men over the age of 45, but also one of the least discussed by those who might become one of the 180,000 new cases diagnosed each year. (HBBMS)

techniques. One of only a handful of such centers in the world, Bayview's facility quickly became a destination for physicians from around the globe who wanted to learn about the latest orthopedic implants, instrumentation and surgical procedures from the Bayview doctors who were pioneering them. Engineers in particular benefited from their experiences at the center, where they could step away from the engineering lab to see surgery first-hand and to watch real-life applications of the equipment they have developed.[23]

The nuclear medicine department at Bayview became one of the first in the region to use positron emission tomography, or PET, a completely noninvasive imaging tool, to detect disease on a cellular level. John Petronis, Bayview's director of nuclear medicine, told *Bayview News* that PET possessed the potential to change the face of medicine with its ability to capture images of working cells and detect disease through abnormalities in the way the cells are functioning, even before changes in body structure, such as tumors, are visible.[24]

A PET scan machine, resembling an open, nonconstricting MRI device, provides a painless look deep inside a patient's body. The patient is given an injection of small amounts of radioactive material attached to a substance familiar to the body, such as sugar. As the patient's body absorbs the sugar normally, the radioactive material "goes along for the ride," as *Bayview News* put it, illuminating the body cells for PET to photograph. The images the machine makes are saved on a computer for a physician to examine for suspicious signs.[25]

Although the technology behind PET was more than 20 years old, it had been used for research, "locked in the laboratory," Petronis said, because of its high cost. When Medicare rules changed late in 2000, covering use of PET for diagnostic purposes, Bayview pioneered its use in patient care to check for early signs of six forms of cancer: lung, colorectal, lymphoma, melanoma, esophageal, and head and neck.[26]

The nationwide movement to adopt the "hospitalist" approach to acute care practice involves employing specialists to focus on a patient's hospital or subacute care from the time of admission to the time of discharge. As the movement grew in the early 2000s, Hopkins Bayview adopted the hospitalist philosophy in its Collaborative Inpatient Medicine Service (CIMS). CIMS brings together nurse practitioners, physician assistants and hospitalists to improve access to services, enhance patient care and provide cost-effective treatment. It ensures continuity and a multidisciplinary approach to the care of the increasing number of inpatients on the general medicine floor of the Francis Scott Key Pavilion, which now bears the name "Zieve Medical Unit" in honor of Philip Zieve's decades of service to the hospital.[27]

The Children's Medical Practice at Hopkins Bayview, under chief of pediatrics Michael Crocetti, offered the atmosphere of a neighborhood pediatric office enhanced with the presence of leading practitioners in their fields. The Children's Center provided extensive specialty services in addition to general pediatric care: Jean Kan headed the pediatric cardiology clinic; Anil Darbari treated children with digestive ailments in the pediatric gastroenterology and motility clinic; surgeon Charles Paidas' pediatric surgery clinic provided comprehensive care for young patients' surgery problems; and Lauren Janson offered complete evaluations of children with development delays or learning disabilities.[28]

Research continued to be a significant undertaking at Hopkins Bayview. The hospital's decades-long pre-eminence in gerontology was continued by the Division of Geriatrics and Gerontology's lead role in identifying changes in the body that put some seniors at greater risk for frailty, an age-related physiological vulnerability to medical illness and injury. A study by Jeremy Walston of 60 individuals (part of a group of 392 screened) found a link between geriatric frailty and an individual's personal biology. The research revealed that the frail elderly have higher markers of inflammation compared to the nonfrail elderly, as well as lower levels of certain hormones that help maintain muscle strength. Walston's findings may lead to new treatments and preventive strategies for

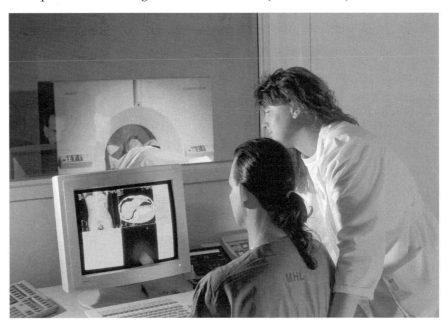

A CT scan is closely observed by **Harvey Brice,** seated, a radiology service technician, and **Stephanie Schluderberg,** a radiology technician. (Mike Ciesielski)

the 8 percent of the population over the age of 70 who are frail and the 50 percent who have some symptoms indicating they are likely to become frail.[29] The new Older American Independence Center, part of the Johns Hopkins Center on Aging and Health and the Johns Hopkins Bloomberg School of Public Health, adjacent to Hopkins Hospital and the school of medicine, undertook to expand on Walston's findings.[30]

Beyond Bayview's main campus, the community centers operated by or affiliated with the Hopkins Bayview Physicians practice group were significantly upgraded and expanded. The old Northpoint Medical Center was closed in 2000 after 15 years of service, and its general medicine providers moved to Johns Hopkins at Merritt Park (operated by Johns Hopkins Community Physicians) and Johns Hopkins at Greater Dundalk, which had undergone $1.1 million in renovations.[31] The new, 50,000-square-foot Johns Hopkins at White Marsh Center opened by Hopkins Community Physicians in 2000 on 3.85 acres northeast of Bayview offered Ob/Gyn services, as well as primary care services in adult medicine, geriatrics and pediatrics; specialty care in cardiology, dermatology, general surgery, plastic surgery, ophthalmology, otolaryngology, orthopedic surgery, urology and podiatry to patients from Bel Air, Perry Hall and White Marsh. The two-story facility also housed eye care services and an optical shop operated by Hopkins' Wilmer Eye Institute, laboratory services performed by staff from The Johns Hopkins Hospital Department of Pathology and Laboratory Medicine, as well as radiological testing provided by American Radiology Services.[32]

ElderPlus, a demonstration program created in 1996 to provide community-based care for elderly individuals who wished to avoid placement in a nursing home, was granted permanent provider status in 2002 by the U.S. Centers for Medicare & Medical Services (CMS) and Maryland's Department of Health and Mental Hygiene. ElderPlus thus became the first provider of such services in Maryland to be given permanent status by the federal Program of All-Inclusive Care for the Elderly (PACE) and among the first in the country to win CMS approval. In its first seven years of operation, the number of participants served by ElderPlus rose from 30 to 150 by the year 2003. "This is a program that's just going to grow, because there are not enough nursing home beds, anywhere, to support all the people who will need them," Greg Schaffer observed.[33]

Responding to the needs of a burgeoning Hispanic population in Bayview's service area, the hospital began on-site Spanish classes in 2003 for Ob/Gyn, pediatrics and the neonatal intensive care unit (NICU) staff, as well as Community Care-A-Van personnel and members of the admitting, mail services, clinical nutrition and public affairs offices. Additional Spanish interpreters also were hired, and educational materials, patient menus and patient rights forms were translated into Spanish. "We hope these classes will make employees more comfortable dealing with Hispanic

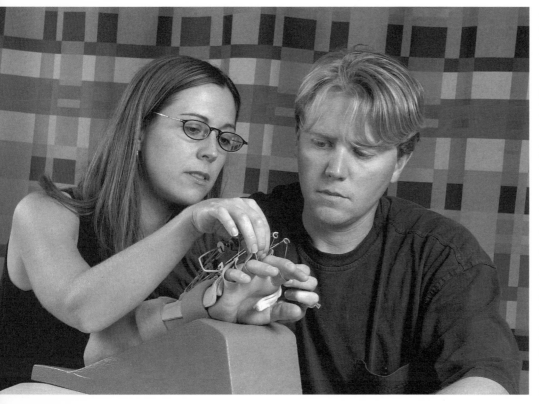

Rehabilitation services at Hopkins Bayview, which opened newly renovated facilities in 2002, offers hand therapy among its 15 specialties, including occupational therapy, physical therapy and speech language pathology services. It treats nearly 500 new outpatients and 1,000 new inpatients every month. Each patient receives individual attention directed by a team of highly skilled, compassionate therapists and physicians. **(HBBMS)**

patients and families," Cathy Mazzotta, director of training and development, told *Dome,* the monthly newspaper of Hopkins Medicine. "Even if all they can say in Spanish is 'Good morning' or 'Don't cry,' it will mean a lot."[34]

Bayview's outreach efforts were not restricted to its off-campus medical centers and health initiatives. Since becoming Bayview's president, Schaffer had spearheaded the hospital's community activities, aimed at demonstrating that Bayview's concerns extended to the neighborhoods where its patients live. He served as chairman of the Southeast Community Development Corporation and secretary of the Greektown Community Development Corporation. He also is a life board member of the Maryland Chapter of the Red Cross, for which he directs periodic blood drives at Bayview that collect more than 1,000 units of blood annually. "How goes the hospital, so goes the community," Schaffer told *Bayview News.* "That's because Bayview comprises a huge part of its community. We're a $300 million-plus operation that employs more than 5,200 people on campus and 3,000 at the Medical Center alone."[35]

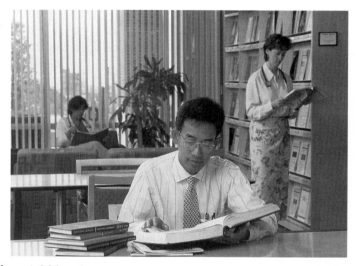

The Harrison Library at the Johns Hopkins Bayview Medical Center assists scholars and researchers by providing the latest medical information and periodicals. The library, which houses 15,000 volumes and 340 medical and professional journals, is named after Harold Harrison, chief of pediatrics at Baltimore City Hospitals from 1945 to 1975. (HBBMS)

The benefits Bayview brought to its community were not measured merely in good intentions and payrolls. Major funding initiatives were involved, too. By 2001, the sums expended on community benefits—including more than $3 million in research, $8 million in medical education, $21.7 million in charity care, and tens of thousands in subsidized programs—totaled $25,329,813.[36]

Bayview's doctors even lent their expertise to the creatures inhabiting the National Aquarium in Baltimore. They also inspired a work of literature.

John Carbone, former chief of the Division of Spine Surgery at Bayview, offered to treat a variety of unusual patients including sea turtles, dolphins and monkeys at the Aquarium. He performed operations to treat an infected tail fin on an 850-pound, 11-foot-long, bottle-nosed dolphin named Bo; two endangered Kemp's Ridley sea turtles (one had a bacterial infection in its elbow; the other had a tumor in its shoulder) and a Gold Lion Tamarin monkey with a broken leg.[37]

The work of the Baltimore Regional Burn Center at Bayview prompted Priscilla Cummings, who got her introduction to the center as a reporter for *Baltimore* magazine, to write *A Face First,* published in 2001 by Dutton's Children's Books. The story of a 12-year-old girl from Maryland's Eastern Shore who is treated at Bayview for severe burns suffered in an automobile accident, *A Face First* condenses the complex procedures at the Burn Center and the medical terminology of its specialists into language a youngster can understand. It relates the compelling story of how its main character overcomes her fears and begins her long journey on the road to recovery.[38]

Recognition of Bayview's excellence continued to be bestowed, both by the community and by those on its campus. In 2003, John R. Burton's 35 years of

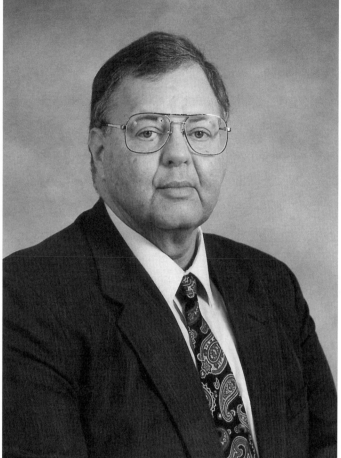

L. Kenneth Grabill II, master of Hopkins Bayview's financial operations since 1982, when Hopkins Hospital began managing the old City Hospitals under a municipal contract, has kept the books in the black for two decades. (HBBMS)

leadership of the Hopkins Bayview's geriatrics program was recognized when the medical center's geriatrics building was named the John R. Burton Pavilion in his honor. "Our patients and trainees are the beneficiaries of Burton's vision," Ron Peterson said at the unveiling ceremony.[39] (A few months later, the Geriatrics Center located in the Burton Pavilion was renamed the Johns Hopkins Bayview Care Center, reflecting the fact that its broad range of continuing care services had expanded well beyond its nursing home origins.[40])

Burton also was among 13 Bayview physicians named in *Baltimore* magazine's 2003 survey of the region's "Top Docs." After surveying thousands of area physicians about whom they considered the best in various specialties, the magazine reported that Bayview's doctors were deemed superior in many disciplines. In addition to Burton in geriatric medicine, the magazine named Tom Finucane in geriatrics, Frederick Sieber in anesthesiology, Patrick Murphy in infectious diseases, Randy Barker and Bruce Leff in internal medicine, Alessandro Olivi in neurological surgery, Geoff Cundiff and George Huggins in Ob/Gyn, Robert Weinberg in ophthalmology, Barbara De Lateur in physical medicine and rehabilitation, Robert Wise in pulmonary and critical care, and Frederick Eckhauser in surgery.[41]

The Division of Rheumatology received more than $1.75 million in pledges from grateful patients, and John Stone, director of the Johns Hopkins Vasculitis Center and deputy director for clinical research for the Department of Medicine, was named chairman of the International Network for the Study of Systemic Vasculitis.[42]

Bayview News, mailed by the hospital to 150,000 community members in its primary and secondary market areas, was honored by the Maryland Society of Health Care Marketing and Public Relations as first in its class for community newsletters.[43]

Constant as Bayview's accomplishments were, its leadership, inevitably, began to change. Early in 2003, Philip Zieve announced his retirement as vice president of medical affairs and was succeeded by Richard D. Bennett, executive medical director of the Johns Hopkins Geriatrics Center.[44] Bennett brought a wealth of experience as a clinician, researcher, educator and program-builder to his new position. As executive medical director of the Geriatrics Center, he had led a variety of clinical programs, many of which became national models of care. He directed the fellowship training program in geriatric medicine, overseeing and mentoring one of the largest groups of clinical and research geriatrics fellows in the country. He is active statewide and nationally in developing new approaches to the delivery of health care for older adults.[45]

By the end of fiscal year 2003, Johns Hopkins Bayview Medical Center had experienced growth in every facet of its operations (except, fortunately, the average patient's length of stay). Inpatient admissions rose from 18,757 in 2002 to 19,684 in 2003; outpatient visits jumped from 90,953 to 97,948; emergency department visits went up from 48,109 to 49,746; and geriatrics admissions increased from 1,249 to 1,271. The average length of stay declined from 4.61 days to 4.58.[46] The community psychiatry program handled a remarkable total of 113,636 visits.[47]

Indeed, Hopkins Bayview's 20-year record of service growth from 1984 to 2003 is astounding: Outpatient clinic visits grew by 80 percent; inpatient admissions rose 86 percent; total surgical procedures soared 87 percent; emergency room visits increased 52 percent. More than 1,800 employees were added to the payroll.[48]

Kenneth Grabill, still the master of Bayview's financial operation after more than 20 years, helped keep its books in the black for a second consecutive decade. In 2003, he coordinated and negotiated a full rate application with the state's Health Services Cost Review Commission (HSCRC), obtaining an overall 3.5 percent increase to Bayview's rates and charging authority. The higher compensation benefited the medical center's fiscal 2003 budget by approximately $1.59 million in net revenues and is expected to benefit future years' net revenues by about $7.5 million.[49]

As the 20th anniversary of Johns Hopkins' acquisition of the old City Hospitals approached, trustee Robert D.H. Harvey observed proudly that Hopkins Bayview had become "really the newest medical hospital on the whole Baltimore front, having been built and put into working order well after the other hospitals were."[50] In reviewing the hospital's astonishing transformation, *Dome* marked the impending milestone by asking, "What will Bayview do for an encore?"[51]

Greg Schaffer envisions a redoubling of efforts to provide services to the constantly increasing number of patients within the space that Bayview presently has available, as well as an expansion of the number of acute care beds. This may be achieved either by renovating the old City Hospitals' A Building, which is part of the acute care hospital, or expanding the Francis Scott Key Pavilion itself.[52] Research space also is at a premium. The National Institutes of Health plans to erect a mammoth, 550,000-square-foot building for several of its existing programs on the campus, including the National

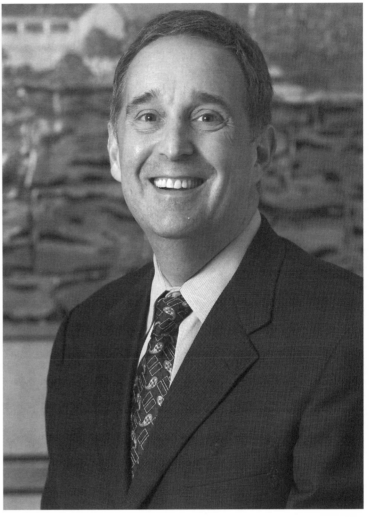

Richard D. Bennett, a clinician, researcher, educator and executive medical director of the Johns Hopkins Geriatrics Center, succeeded Philip Zieve as vice president of medical affairs at Hopkins Bayview in 2003. (Kevin Weber)

Institute on Drug Abuse and National Institute on Aging's Gerontology Research Center.[53] That could open additional research space on campus for Hopkins Bayview's scientists.

The merger of the faculty practices prompted Frank Frassica, director of orthopedic surgery for the School of Medicine and Hopkins Hospital, and his counterpart at Bayview, the late James Wenz, to concentrate the orthopedic surgery faculty and programs at Bayview, which, they decided, was the campus best suited to handle them. They created the multidisciplinary Musculoskeletal Institute at Bayview focusing on geriatric orthopedics. With the Geriatrics (now Care) Center and the National Institute on Aging already there, Bayview was a natural site for the Musculoskeletal Institute.[54] As another consequence of the faculty merger, David Hellmann was able to expand every part of the rheumatology program at Bayview. Such treatment programs as the Rheumatoid Arthritis Center, headed by Joan Bathon; the Vasculitis Center, headed by John Stone; and the Scleroderma Center, headed by Frederick Wigley, "didn't have enough space at Hopkins Hospital to flourish," Hellmann told *Change,* the Johns Hopkins Medicine biweekly newsletter. "Rheumatology Chief Antony Rosen made them happen here [at Bayview], and they've become integral parts of the Musculoskeletal Institute."[55]

Developments like these herald even more collaboration with The Johns Hopkins Hospital in the future. "We're far more collaborative now," Schaffer told *Dome.* "Department by department, everyone is really focused on the importance of having these two hospitals compliment each other." Judy Reitz forecasts that clinical operations at Bayview and at Hopkins Hospital eventually will be merged completely, and that from an administrative perspective, the two entities will move closer and closer to having a common financial bottom line.[56]

"Do I think there is a point where there is a single merged entity? I don't know that," Reitz says. "It would depend on the most strategic and positive thing to do. At this moment in time, we have decided that to operate two autonomous corporations is the best way to respond to this marketplace. Should that shift in mission or environment occur, we will be ideally situated in order to seamlessly move in that direction."[57]

Ron Peterson, with the unique perspective on both institutions gained from having been president of each, is certain that Bayview will not only prosper but endure. "Bayview will become an increasingly important contributor to the tripartite mission of Johns Hopkins Medicine without becoming a clone of The Johns Hopkins Hospital," Peterson says.[58] "No matter what the future may portend, in terms of corporate structural modification, it is my belief that Bayview will continue to always enjoy its own personality.

"As such, Bayview will carry on its longstanding tradition of serving the citizens of Southeast Baltimore and beyond with the best possible contemporary health care services as a proud member of Johns Hopkins Medicine."[59]

Hopkins Bayview has proven enormously adept at addressing changes in the environment over the past two centuries. Its story "reflects the changes in the management of hospitals and the way hospitals relate to the community over the past 200 years, and it reflects the changes in medical education during that time as well," says Philip Zieve, a perceptive participant in and observer of those changes for more than 45 years.[60]

Bayview is "an institution that has managed to stay alive, despite all these environmental changes," Zieve says. "To do that, you have to have a special genetic makeup. When the environment changes is when organisms die; and the ones that survive have to have the capability to respond to changes in the environment," Zieve observes. "And I think we have."[61]

NOTES

Chapter One

1 Jacques Kelly, draft history (1998; unpublished manuscript on file at the Johns Hopkins Bayview Medical Center's Office of Public Affairs); Susan Ellery Greene, *Baltimore: An Illustrated History*, (Woodland Hills, Calif.: Windsor Publications, 1980), 28.

2 Parker J. McMillin, "Baltimore City Hospitals," *Maryland State Medical Journal* 4(12), Dec. 1955, 748-758 (hereinafter referred to as "McMillin").

3 McMillin.

4 McMillin says 1776; Douglas Carroll, M.D., "History of Baltimore City Hospitals," *Maryland State Medical Journal*, v. 15, 1966 (hereafter referred to as "Carroll") 2, says 1774.

5 Respective Web sites: http://www.phila.gov/health/history/parts/part_5.htm;
http://www.med.nyu.edu/Bellevue/;
http://www.lsuhsc.edu/hcsd/mclno/.

6 Carroll, *op. cit.*

7 Kelly; Carroll, 6.

8 Carroll, 2; Kelly; Robert J. Brugger, *Maryland: A Middle Temperament, 1634-1980* (Baltimore: Johns Hopkins University Press, 1988) 141;
http://physics.bu.edu/~redner/projects/population/cities/baltimore.html. Baltimore would become the country's second largest city in 1830, with 80,620 residents, compared to New York's 202,589.

9 Carroll, 3, 5.

10 *Ibid.*, 5.

11 http://www.redwoodlibrary.org/notables/waterhouse.htm.

12 Carroll; W.E. Earle, "Pox Americana," *The City Paper*, Feb. 5, 2003, 21.

13 Carroll, 3, fig. 2.

14 *Ibid.*, 6.

15 *Ibid.*, 7-8.

16 Carroll, 6-8; McMillin, 750; Kelly.

17 Carroll, 11; Kelly.

18 Kelly.

19 Carroll, 8, 10.

20 *Ibid.*, 17.

21 *Ibid.*, 8.

22 *Ibid.*, 9.

23 *Ibid.*, 8, 10.

24 *Ibid.*, 15.

25 *Ibid.*, 37.

26 *Ibid.*, 17.

27 A.M. Shipley, M.D. and O.C. Brantigan, M.D., "The Surgical Service of Baltimore City Hospitals," *Maryland State Medical Journal* 4(12), Dec. 1955, 765.

28 Carroll, 18-19; McMillin, 750; Kelly.

29 Carroll, 18; Kelly.

30 McMillin, 751.

31 George S. Mirick, "Medical Department of the Baltimore City Hospitals," *Maryland State Medical Journal* 4(12), Dec. 1955, 758-759.

32 Carroll, 18.

33 *Ibid.*, 21-22; A. McGehee Harvey, Gert H. Brieger, Susan L. Abrams, and Victor A. McKusick, *A Model of Its Kind: A Centennial History of Medicine at Johns Hopkins* (Baltimore: Johns Hopkins University Press, 1989), 20.

34 Carroll, 18, 21; Mirick, *Maryland State Medical Journal* 4(12), Dec. 1955, 759.

35 Baltimore City Hospitals, *The Record* II(5), Mar. 1960, 3.

36 *The Record*, II(5), Mar. 1960, 3; .

37 *Maryland State Medical Journal* 22(11), Nov. 1973, 53.

38 Carroll, 21.

39 *Ibid.*

40 "History of Tuberculosis Division, Baltimore City Hospitals," *Maryland State Medical Journal* 4(12), Dec. 1955, 771.

41 Mirick, *Maryland State Medical Journal* 4(12), Dec. 1955, 759.

42 Carroll, 23.

43 Karen Harrop, "Nursing History" draft history, unpublished manuscript on file at the Johns Hopkins Bayview Medical Center's Office of Public Affairs (n.d.), 2.

44 McMillin, 751; Carroll, 23.

45 Kelly.

46 P. Stewart Macaulay, "Addition to Be Dedicated Today...," *The Sun*, Apr. 28, 1935; Carroll, 40.

47 Edmund G. Beacham, *Maryland State Medical Journal*, 4 (12), Dec. 1955, 771-772.

48 *Maryland State Medical Journal*, 4(12), portraits and dates on cover, 765; Carroll, 24-25.

49 *Maryland State Medical Journal*, *op. cit*, 759; Carroll, 24-25; Harry F. Dowling, *City Hospitals: The Undercare of the Underprivileged* (Cambridge, MA: Harvard University Press, 1982), 115.

50 Dowling, *City Hospitals*, 115.

51 *Ibid.*, 115 and 125-126. In 1955, members of the surgery unit opposed the University of Maryland's nominee as surgeon in chief and urged the appointment of Mark M. Ravitch, a highly regarded Hopkins-trained surgeon. The University of Maryland, resentful of this move despite Ravitch's acknowledged success reinvigorating the surgical service, gradually ended its ties to City Hospitals.

52 Mirick, *Maryland State Medical Journal*, 4(12) Dec. 1955, 760; Carroll, 25.

53 Carroll, 25-26; *Maryland State Medical Journal* 4(12), Dec. 1955, 772.

54 Carroll, 26; *Maryland State Medical Journal* 4(12), Dec. 1955, 781.

55 Mark S. Watson, "The Regeneration of Bay View," *The Sun*, June 28, 1931. Watson later became a renowned military correspondent; the Pentagon's briefing room is named in his honor.

56 C. Holmes Boyd, "Pride In Our Past," *The Record* 11(5), Mar. 1960, 2.

57 Phillip Zieve speech, FSK Pavilion dedication, Apr. 26, 1994.

58 "Longan Applies for Retirement," Archives Box 39, Fold #1, Mat #14. *The Sun* (?), (date?) page (?); Watson, "The Regeneration of Bay View."

59 "Longan Applies for Retirement."

60 Watson, "The Regeneration of Bay View;" "Nursing History," 4; "Logan Applies for Retirement."

61 "Nursing History;" interview with Philip Zieve, M.D., May 13, 2003 (hereinafter referred to as "Zieve int. 5/13/03").

62 Carroll, 26.

63 *Ibid.*

64 Watson, "The Regeneration of Bay View;" "City Hospitals Survey Urged by Col. Longan," *The Sun*, Oct. 19, 1929; *The Record* I(3), Nov.-Dec. 1958, 1.

65 "New Facilities for Bay View," *The Sun*, Apr. 28, 1935; *Maryland State Medical Journal*, Dec. 1955, 760; Carroll, 27.

66 *The Record*, Nov-Dec. 1958, 1-2.

67 "New Facilities for Bay View," *The Sun*, Apr. 28, 1935; Carroll, 28-29.

68 *Maryland State Medical Journal* Dec. 1955, McMillin, 51; Carroll, 27.

69 Carroll, 26, 28.

70 Carroll, 27; *Maryland State Medical Journal* Dec. 1955; Mirick, 760-61.

71 McMillin, 751; Carroll, 28; *Maryland State Medical Journal* 22(11) Nov. 1973, 55; E.G. Beacham, M.D., "Geriatrics in Maryland: Challenges for the Eighties," *Maryland State Medical Journal* 32(9), Sept. 1983, 686.

72 "Nursing History," 6.

73 *The Record*, I(3), Nov.-Dec. 1958, McMillin, 2.

74 "Nursing History," 7.

75 Carroll, 28-29.

76 *Ibid.*, 29.

77 *Ibid.*

78 *Ibid.*, 31.
79 "Profiles," *The Record* III(2), Sept. 1960, 3.
80 Slide presentation, 2001, on City Hospital/Bayview highlights.
81 Mirick, *Maryland State Medical Journal* 4(12), Dec. 1955, 761.
82 Author interview with Philip Zieve, May 13, 2003 (hereinafter "Zieve int. 5/13/03").
83 *Ibid.*
84 *Maryland State Medical Journal* 4(12) Dec. 1955, McMillin, 752-753.
85 "City Hospitals Head to Retire," *The Sun*, Feb. 18, 1959.
86 Author interview with Chester W. Schmidt Jr., May 23, 2003 (hereinafter "Schmidt int.").
87 "Dr. Schmidt Appointed Chief of Psychiatry," *The Pillbox*, Baltimore City Hospitals, 15(14), Oct. 1, 1972, 1; "Dr. Schmidt to Head CPPA," *The Pillbox*, 20(5), Nov. 18, 1977, 1.
88 Weldon Wallace, "City Hospitals Transformed By Staff In Last 15 Years," *The Sun*, July 1, 1960.
89 *Maryland State Medical Journal*, 22(11) Nov. 1973, 45-46.
90 Zieve int. 5/13/03.
91 "Mr. McMillin Leaves," *The Sun* (unsigned editorial), Feb. 21, 1959.
92 Carroll, 36.
93 Nisha Chibber Chandra, M.D., letter to Sue Davis, Jan. 18, 1995; "Peter Safar," *The Record*, III(4), Jan. 1961, 1; Anita Srikameswaran, "Dr. Peter Safar, Renowned Pitt physician called 'father of CPR,'" *Pittsburgh Post-Gazette*, Aug. 5, 2003.
94 Carroll, 32; *Maryland State Medical Journal*, 22 (11) Nov. 1973, 52.
95 *Maryland State Medical Journal*, 22(11) Nov. 1973, 55.
96 Carroll, 34.
97 *Maryland State Medical Journal* 22(11), Nov. 1973, 56; Zieve speech at dedication ceremony for Francis Scott Key Pavilion, Apr. 27, 1994.
98 Carroll, 35; *The Record* VIII(3), Dec. 1965, 4; Zieve int. 5/13/03
99 Zieve int., 5/13/03.
100 *The Record* VIII(3), Dec. 1965, 4.
101 Carroll, 44; *Maryland State Medical Journal* 22(11), Nov. 1973, 56-57.
102 *Maryland State Medical Journal* 22(11), Nov. 1973, 46.
103 Bayview Archives, Box 22; Folder 1, Mat. #4; "Maryland's First Burn Unit Opens Here," *The Record* XI(2), January 1969, 1-2.
104 *Kiwanis Magazine*, Feb. 1994, "Burn center snuffs pains from flames," 46; *Capital Builder*, Oct. 1994, photo cutline.
105 Peggy Radawich, "1st Kidney Swap Made Here," *The News American*, Nov. 2, 1968; Mohammed Rauf Jr., "New Heart 'Pacemaker' Rechargeable Under Skin," *The News American*, Nov. 17, 1969.
106 *Maryland State Medical Journal* 22(11), Nov. 1973, 56-57; *The Pillbox*, 13(10), "Division of Chronic Medical Care," Nov. 27, 1970.
107 *Maryland State Medical Journal*, 22(11) Nov. 1973, 57.
108 Zieve int. 5/13/03; Schmidt int.
109 Zieve int. 5/13/03.
110 Schmidt int.
111 Drs. Chester W. Schmidt Jr., Philip D. Zieve, and Burton C. D'Lugoff, "A Practice Plan in a Municipal Teaching Hospital: A Model for the Funding of Clinical Faculty," *New England Journal of Medicine*, 304(5):263 (1981); Mary Knudson, "Physicians Group is a Power at City Hospitals," *The Sun*, Aug. 28, 1977; *Maryland State*

Medical Journal 22(11), Nov. 1973, 48.
112 *Maryland State Medical Journal*, 22(11) Nov. 1973, 46; CPPA Annual Report, 1976; *Change*, Dec. 12, 2001, "The Little Giant," *CPA News*, 5; Zieve int. 5/13/03.
113 Zieve int. 5/13/03; Schmidt int.
114 CPPA Annual Report, 1976.
115 Knudson, "Physicians group is a power at City Hospitals."
116 *Ibid.*
117 *Change* 5(20), Dec. 12, 2001, 5; Zieve int. 5/13/03.
118 Knudson, "Physicians group is a power at City Hospitals;" "Baltimore City Hospitals: Third Century of Service" (booklet), 1973.
119 "Baltimore City Hospitals: Third Century of Service;" Candy York, "The Almshouse of 1773 Still Serves the Needs of 1973's Baltimoreans," *The News American*, Dec. 28, 1973, B1.
120 *Ibid.*
121 *Congressional Record*, 119(169), Nov. 6, 1973, "Baltimore City Hospitals' Bicentennial," Hon. Paul S. Sarbanes of Maryland in the House of Representatives; Mayor William Donald Schaefer, Proclamation, Oct. 17, 1973; "Baltimore City Hospitals: Third Century of Service," 1973, section heading: "Baltimore City Hospitals Tomorrow."
122 "Heal Thyself," *The Evening Sun*, (unsigned editorial), Nov. 20, 1975; "Doctor, Heal Thy Hospital," *The Sun* (unsigned editorial), Oct. 26, 1981.

Chapter Two

1 E.G. Beacham, M.D., D.G. Carroll, M.D. and F.G. Hubbard, "Toward a Third Century of Progress," *Maryland State Medical Journal* 22(11), Nov. 1973, 45-47.
2 Richard Ben Cramer, "City Hospitals losing millions in fiscal tangle," *The Sun*, Nov. 20, 1975, 11.
3 Schmidt int.
4 *Ibid.*
5 Gwen Ifill, "Hospital change cost—$2 million," *The Evening Sun*, Mar. 16, 1982.
6 Cramer, "City Hospitals losing millions in fiscal tangle."
7 *Ibid.*
8 *Ibid.*
9 *The Sun*, "City Hospitals director resigns," July 1, 1976.
10 "Heal Thyself," *The Evening Sun*.
11 Jeff Valentine, "City Hospitals ... Nearing 'Anarchy,'" *The Evening Sun*, Mar. 3, 1977, 1.
12 Valentine, *op.cit.*; Drew Marcks, "City Hospitals In 'Anarchy,'" *The News American*, Mar. 3, 1977, City & Counties section, 1.
13 *Ibid.*
14 "Letter to All Employees," *The Pillbox* 20(2), Mar. 11, 1977.
15 Marcks, "Union Defends Employes Rapped At City Hospitals," *The News American*, Mar. 4, 1977, City & Counties section, 1.
16 Valentine, "Angry City Hospitals Employes Deny Reports of 'Anarchy' At Facility," *The Evening Sun*, Mar. 4, 1977, 1.
17 *Ibid.*
18 Author's interview with Burton D'Lugoff, Aug. 18, 2003 (hereinafter "D'Lugoff int.").
19 G. Jefferson Price 3rd, "Hospitals Firings Expected; 11 administrative posts vacant at city facility," *The Sun*, Mar. 4, 1977.
20 Zieve int. 5/13/03.
21 *The Evening Sun*, Mar. 4, 1977, editorial page; Mar. 3, 1977, editorial page.
22 History of Philadelphia Hospitals Web site,

http://www.phila.gov/health/history/parts/part_5.htm; Robert Heyssel, oral history interview with Mame Warren, Nov. 28, 2000, 56, Johns Hopkins Medicine Archives (hereinafter referred to as "Heyssel").
23 Heyssel, 56; Built St. Louis Web site, http://www.builtstlouis.net/crumble01.html; Michael R. Allen (local St. Louis historian) Web site, http://www.spintechmag.com/allen/stlouis/visithosp.htm.
24 Zieve int. 5/13/03.
25 *The Sun*, "City names Hospitals director," Mar. 18, 1977.
26 CPPA: Annual Report of the Chesapeake Physicians Professional Association, 1977; Mary Knudson, "Physicians group is a power at City Hospitals," *The Sun*, Aug. 8, 1977; "Staff's Aim: Fill Empty Beds At City Hospital," Jeff Valentine, Dec. 28, 1978; "Chesapeake Physicians Has Critics," *The Evening Sun*, Dec. 29, 1978.
27 Jeff Valentine, "Staff's Aim: Fill Empty Beds at City Hospital," *The Evening Sun*, Dec. 28, 1978.
28 D'Lugoff int.; CPPA Annual Reports, 1976 and 1977.
29 Interview with Ron Peterson, Nov. 1, 2003; e-mail from Philip Zieve, Nov. 20, 2003; CareFirst Blue Cross, James P. Day, Apr, 12, 2004.
30 CPPA Annual Report, 1976.
31 D'Lugoff int.
32 *Ibid.*
33 *Ibid.*
34 Chester W. Schmidt Jr.; Philip D. Zieve; Burton C. D'Lugoff, "A Practice Plan in a Municipal Teaching Hospital: A Model for the Funding of Clinical Faculty," *New England Journal of Medicine* 304(5), Jan. 29, 1981.
35 Jay Spry, "Russell, 'left in dark,' quits City Hospitals," *The Sun*, July 7, 1982; *The Evening Sun*, "City Hospital executive director quits," July 7, 1982.
36 Nick Yengich, "Head of hospital in Boston first choice for top job at City," *The Evening Sun*, Oct. 22, 1981; *The Sun*, "Doctor, Heal Thy Hospital," (unsigned editorial), Oct. 26, 1981.
37 Sue Miller, "City Hospital seeks new doctors, new patients," *The Evening Sun*, June 17, 1981.
38 William Donald Schaefer speech, Apr. 26, 1994, at opening of the Francis Scott Key Pavilion at Johns Hopkins Bayview Medical Center (hereinafter "Schaefer speech").
39 Heyssel oral history, 54; HCA Web site, History section, http://www.hcahealthcare.com/CustomPage.aspx?guidC ustomContentID=D52E3835-8DB5-4137-9940-18BDDCB211E2; http://www.scripophily.net/ammedin-inc.html (Stock certificate for AMI, with brief history of firm, now part of American Medical Holdings); Schmidt int.
40 Author's interview with Ron Peterson, Feb. 24, 2003 (hereinafter "Peterson Int. 2/24/03").
41 Author's interview with Edward Halle, May 20, 2003, (hereinafter "Halle int.").
42 *The Sun*, "Hopkins Hospital may bid to manage City Hospitals," Sept. 10, 1981, C1.
43 Author's interview with Judith Reitz, Aug. 12, 2003 (hereinafter "Reitz int.").
44 *Ibid*; e-mail from Reitz to author, Aug. 19, 2003, with notes from Sept. 1981 report.
45 *Ibid.*
46 *The Sun*, "Hopkins Hospital may bid to manage City Hospitals."
47 Zieve int. 5/13/03.
48 Schmidt int.
49 Robert Heyssel, voice on tribute tape for Ronald Peterson (undated).
50 Heyssel oral history 50-51, 54.
51 *Ibid.*, 54.
52 *Ibid.*

53 Peterson int. 2/24/03.

54 Heyssel oral history, 55.

55 Minutes, Joint Committee of Trustees, JHU/JHH, Apr. 5, 1982; Minutes of Budget and Operations Committee, Apr. 19, 1982; Minutes of The Johns Hopkins Hospital Board of Trustees Executive Session, May 4, 1982.

56 Minutes of The Johns Hopkins Hospital Board of Trustees, Executive Session, May 4, 1982.

57 Maury Macht, "Hospitals to discuss takeover; Hopkins trustees OK talks with city," *The News American*, May 5, 1982.

58 Johns Hopkins Hospital Board of Trustees minutes, May 4, 1982.

59 Macht, "Hospitals to discuss takeover; Hopkins trustees OK talks with city;" Cynthia Skove, "Hopkins nears agreement to take over City Hospitals," *The News American*, Nov. 29, 1983, 1A and 6A; Spry, "Russell 'left in the dark'…," *The Sun*; "City Hospital executive director quits, *The Evening Sun*, both July 7, 1982.

60 *The Evening Sun* July 7, 1982; A. Yvonne Russell, M.D., letter to Cleve Laub Jr., administrator of Francis Scott Key Medical Center, Aug. 16, 1988.

61 *The Sun*, July 7, 1982, *op. cit.*

62 Cynthia Skove, "Hopkins nears agreement to take over City Hospitals," *The News American*, Nov. 29, 1983.

63 Heyssel on Peterson tribute tape (undated).

64 Bond application, 1989, "Executive Management" descriptions; author's interview with Ken Grabill, Sept. 25, 2003 (hereinafter "Grabill int. 9/25/03").

65 Author's interview with Bill Ward, Aug. 13, 2003 (hereinafter "Ward int."); Ward e-mail to author, Oct. 13, 2003.

66 Grabill int. 9/25/03.

67 Ward int.

68 Grabill int. 9/25/03.

69 Ronald Peterson, oral history interview with Mame Warren, Mar. 8, 2001, 4-6 (hereinafter "Peterson oral history"); Ward int.

70 Peterson oral history, 6.

71 Author's interviews with Ken Grabill, Sept. 25 and Oct. 1, 2003.

72 "A Few Moments with Ron Peterson," *Keynotes, The Francis Scott Key Medical Center* 3(2), Summer 1987, 17-18.

73 *Ibid.*

74 Schmidt int.

75 Author's interviews with Grabill; Grabill memo to author, Oct. 1, 2003.

76 Grabill int. 9/25/03.

77 *Ibid.*

78 *Ibid.*

79 Heyssel oral history, 54.

80 Minutes of Joint Committee of Trustees, JHU/JHH, Feb. 7, 1983.

81 Peterson int. 2/24/03; Schmidt int.

82 Author's interview with Walter Sondheim, Oct. 22, 2003 (hereinafter "Sondheim int.").

83 Halle int.

84 Minutes of Joint Committee of Trustees of The Johns Hopkins University and Hospital, Mar. 10, 1983.

85 *The News American*, May 5, 1982; Frank D. Roylance and Richard Berke, "City reaches pact to transfer hospital to Hopkins July 1," *The Evening Sun*, Mar. 12, 1984, D1.

86 *The Johns Hopkins Magazine*, June 1984, 47.

87 Peterson int. 2/24/03; Heyssel oral history; *East Baltimore Guide* newspaper, photo caption, May 17, 1984.

88 Heyssel oral history, 54; Peterson int. 2/24/03; *The Johns Hopkins Magazine*, June 1984, 47; *The Evening Sun*, Mar. 12, 1984.

89 Interview with Ron Peterson, July 21, 2003 (here-

inafter "Peterson int. 7/21/03"); Grabill int. 9/25/03.

90 Heyssel oral history, 54.

91 Sondheim int.

92 Charles Benton, speech at groundbreaking for Francis Scott Key Pavilion, Oct. 15, 1991.

93 Peterson int. 7/21/03.

94 Schaefer speech, Apr. 26, 1994.

95 *The News American*, "Hopkins nears agreement … ," Nov. 29, 1983.

96 Frank D. Roylance and Richard Berke, "City reaches pact to transfer hospital to Hopkins July 1," *The Evening Sun*, Mar. 12, 1984.

97 Ron Davis, "Council grill Hopkins, city on shift of hospital," *The Sun*, Apr. 13, 1984, E1-2; Frank D. Roylance, "Hopkins takeover vote due; Council still has questions," *The Evening Sun*, Apr. 13, 1984, D1-2.

98 Heyssel oral history, 55: "It's been rebuilt basically by money generated out there. I mean, Hopkins Hospital itself has guaranteed part of the debt, but I don't believe we put a cent in the place, not initially or now."

99 *Ibid.*

100 Grabill int. 9/25/03.

101 Mark Miller, "City Hospitals sale to Johns Hopkins approved," *The News American*, Apr. 17, 1984, 4A; Frank D. Roylance, "Hospital takeover vote due," *The Evening Sun*, Apr. 13, 1984, D1-2; Ron Davis, "Council grills Hopkins, city on shift of hospital," *The Sun*, Apr. 13, 1984, E1-2.

102 *Ibid.* Two of the 19 members of the City Council were not present for the vote.

103 Zieve int. 5/13/03.

104 *The Evening Sun*, "City Hospital executive director quits," July 7, 1982; *The Evening Sun*, "A fiscal surgeon takes the reins at troubled City Hospital," Sue Miller, Sept. 14, 1982; *The Evening Sun*, "City Hospital seeks new doctors, new patients," June 17, 1981.

105 Dennis O'Shea, personal communication to author (on Ross Jones' role in renaming City Hospitals); Sandy Banisky, "City Hospitals gets new owner—and new name," *The Sun*, July 3, 1984; Deborah I. Greene, "Hospital officials hope new name will cure image," *The Evening Sun*, July 3, 1984, D4.

106 Photos in *The Sun* and *The Evening Sun*, July 3, 1984; Mark Miller, "City Hospitals gets image lift; New name, system to collect debts," *The News American*, July 5, 1984, 12A.

107 *Ibid.*, *The News American*, July 5, 1984.

108 *Ibid.*; Ken Grabill memorandum to author, Oct. 1, 2003; Ward int.

109 Heyssel oral history 55; Ken Grabill memorandum to author, Oct. 1, 2003.

110 Schaefer speech, Apr. 26, 1994.

Chapter Three

1 Harry F. Dowling, M.D., *City Hospitals: The Undercare of the Underprivileged* (Cambridge, MA: Harvard University Press, 1982), 2; The Robert Wood Johnson Foundation Web site, "Report on the Status of Public Hospitals in Major Cities," updated November 2000.

2 *Ibid.*, Robert Wood Johnson Web site.

3 Dowling, *City Hospitals,* 185.

4 *Ibid.*, 177, 185-187.

5 The Johns Hopkins Bayview Medical Center PowerPoint presentation slides, 2001; interview with Carl H. Francioli, Senior Director, Finance, Apr. 16, 2004.

6 FSK press release: "Vice President for Nursing Appointed," Nov. 7, 1984; Johns Hopkins Medicine press release: "Judy Reitz Appointed Executive Vice President and Chief Operating Officer of the Johns Hopkins Hospital," Oct. 12, 1999; bond application,

1989 ("Executive Management" descriptions).

7 *Ibid.*

8 Francis Scott Key Medical Center 1985 Annual Report, 1-2; "Viewpoint," *Keynotes* 1(2), Summer 1985, 1.

9 Author's interview with Zieve, Dec. 17, 2003 (hereinafter "Zieve int. 12/17/03").

10 Peterson int. 7/21/03.

11 *Ibid.*

12 Grabill int. 9/25/03.

13 Author's interview with William McCarthy, April 5, 2004.

14 Author's interview with Francis X. Knott, April 5, 2004.

15 *Keynotes* 1(2) Summer 1985, 1; 1985 Annual Report, 6.

16 *Ibid.*

17 *Ibid.*, 1985 Annual Report, 6.

18 *Keynotes*, 1(2) Summer 1985, 1.

19 Grabill int. 9/25/03.

20 Annual Report, 1985, 7.

21 *Ibid.*, 8.

22 *Ibid.*

23 *Ibid.*, 8-9.

24 *Ibid.*, 9.

25 Peterson int. 7/21/03.

26 Ward int.

27 *Ibid.*

28 *Ibid.*

29 1985 Annual Report, 7.

30 *Keynotes*, 1(2) Summer 1985, 13; Bayview PowerPoint slides, 2001.

31 *Ibid.*, *Keynotes*, 1; Bayview PowerPoint slides.

32 *Ibid.*, *Keynotes.*

33 *Ibid.*, *Keynotes*, 1; author's interview with John Burton, June 11, 2003 (hereinafter "Burton int.").

34 *Keynotes* 1(2) Summer 1985,15.

35 *Ibid.*, *Keynotes* 1(2) Summer 1985, 12.

36 *Keynotes* 1(2) Summer 1985, 12.

37 *Keynotes* 1(2) Summer 1985, 12; revenue bond request to Maryland Health and Higher Education Facilities Authority, July 1, 1990, B14-15.

38 *Keynotes* 1(2) Summer 1985, 12-13.

39 Author's interview with Gayle Johnson Adams, Sept. 12, 2003 (hereinafter "Adams int. 9/12/03").

40 *Ibid.*

41 *Ibid.*

42 *Ibid.*

43 *Ibid.*

44 *Ibid.*; *Keynotes* Summer 1985, 1.

45 *Community News* 1(3), Fall 1989, 4.

46 Annual Report, 1985, 6.

47 Adams int. 9/12/03.

48 Annual Report, 1985, 11; *Keynotes* 3(2), Summer 1987, "A Few Moments with Ron Peterson," 16- 21; "Going, Going, Gone," *Community News* 1(3), Fall 1989, 1-3; revenue bond request to Maryland Health and Higher Education Facilities Authority, July 1, 1990, B14-15.

49 McMillin, "Baltimore City Hospitals," *Maryland State Medical Journal*, 4(12) Dec. 1955; 750-751; Sandy Reckert-Reusing, "What's In a Name?", *Bayviews* 7(1), 5; revenue bond request, July 1, 1990, B14.

50 Ward int.

51 *Maryland State Medical Journal* 4(12), Dec. 1955; Burton int.

52 Revenue bond request.

53 *Keynotes* 3(2) Summer 1987, 18.

54 Grabill int. 9/25 /03.

55 *Ibid.*, 17-18.

56 Ronald Peterson, "Viewpoint," *Keynotes* 2(2), Fall 1986, 2.

57 *Ibid.*, "Introducing … The Johns Hopkins Health

System," 14-15.

58 *Ibid.*, "CMEA Union is Voted Out," 15; press release, "CMEA-Represented Employees AT FSKMC Vote Against Union Representation," May 30, 1986.

59 *Ibid.*

60 *Ibid.*

61 Ward int.

62 Peterson int. 2/24/03.

63 FSK press releases, Mar. 10, 1986, "Baltimore Regional Burn Center Seeks State Appropriation"; [undated] follow-up release draft re: presentation of plaques following 1986 General Assembly; videotapes of Geriatric Center dedication, June 6, 1991; groundbreaking for acute patient care tower, Oct. 15, 1991; FSK Pavilion opening, Apr. 26-27, 1994.

64 Linell Smith, "Physician pushes geriatric reforms," "Day care a step for independence," *The Evening Sun*, March 18, 1988, A1; Lisa G. DeNike, "ElderCall Update," *Keynotes* 3(2), Summer 1987, 22-24; author's telephone interview with Edmund Beacham, Apr. 12, 2004.

65 *Keynotes* 2(2), Fall 1986, 18; slide show presentation on FSK geriatrics, slide # 9.

66 "Bennett Receives Prestigious Geriatrics Award," press release, Feb. 24, 1987; "Andres Receives Prestigious Geriatrics Award," press release, Mar. 20, 1987.

67 "FSKMC to Screen More Than 15,000 Smokers in National Lung Study," press release, Feb. 26, 1987; "FSJMC To Test Nicotine Patch for Smokers," undated press release; *Community News* , "Nicotine Skin Patch Tested at Medical Center," 1(2), Spring 1989.

68 *Keynotes* 3(1) Spring 1987, 17; "Dome Corp. Breaks Ground for Asthma Center," *Keynotes* 3(2) Summer 1987, 44-45.

69 "Dr. Andrew Munster, 67, Burn Center Chief," *The Sun* (obituary), Sept. 30, 2003.

70 *The Banner* 2(13), Jan. 31, 1986; "Maryland Burn Victim Receives First Cultured Skin Graft in Maryland at Baltimore Regional Burn Center," press release, July 20, 1988; "Ceremony Marks Completion of Renovations to Burn Center at FSKMC,"Oct. 21, 1988.

71 "Dr. Andrew Munster, 67, Burn Center Chief," *The Sun*, Sept. 30, 2003.

72 Editorial memorandum, Nov. 4, 1988 for press briefing on groundbreaking; "FSKMC to Break Ground for New Geriatric Center and Phase I Redevelopment," press release, Nov. 10, 1988; *Community News* 1(2), Spring 1989, 1 and 4.

73 "FSKMC to Break Ground for New Geriatric Center and Phase I Redevelopment," press release, Nov. 10, 1988.

74 "Digestive Diseases Staff Opens New Endoscopy Suite," press release Jan. 23, 1989; "FSKMC Pharmacist Wins National Research Award," press release, Feb. 3, 1989; "FSKMC Opens Chemical Dependency Center for Adolescents," Apr. 6, 1989; "$10 Million Grant Establishes Drug Abuse Treatment/Research Unit at FSKMC," press release, Nov. 7, 1989.

75 *Community News* 1(3), Fall 1989, 1 and 4.

76 *Ibid.*, "Former Nurses Residence at FSKMC Slated for Implosion," press release, Aug. 27, 1989.

77 *Community News*, Fall 1989.

78 "Hopkins to Open $45 Million Asthma & Allergy Center in November," draft press release, Nov. 9, 1989.

79 *Ibid.*; Jonathan Bor, "Center aims at mysteries of asthma," *The Sun*, Nov. 19, 1989.

Chapter Four

1 Lisa DeNike, "Redevelopment: Progress and Surprises," *Community News* 2(1), Spring 1990, 4.

2 *Ibid.*

3 *Ibid.*; "New Geriatrics Center Opens in Late Spring," *Community News* 3(1), Spring 1991, 1.

4 Memo from Ken Grabill, Oct, 1, 2003, with accompanying list of "Trend of Revenue over Expenses, Fiscal Years 1985-1995."

5 *Community News* 2(2), Fall 1990, "Bond Sale Paves Way for New Addition," 1; Press release, "Groundbreaking for Key Medical Center Tower," Oct. 4, 1991 .

6 *Community News* 2(2), Fall 1990, "Bond Sale Paves Way for New Addition," 1.

7 Press release, "Center for Burn Reconstruction Opens at FSKMC," Sept. 11, 1990.

8 *Community News* 2(2), Fall 1990, "Community Plays Role In Burn Center Success," 3.

9 *Ibid.*

10 Press Release, "The Johns Hopkins Obesity Center Opens On Hopkins Bayview Research Campus," Sept. 20, 1990; press release, "Center for Occupational and Environmental Health Opens at FSKMC," Feb. 13, 1999.

11 Press release, "Center for Occupational and Environmental Health Opens at FSKMC," Feb. 13, 1991.

12 "DHMH and Francis Scott Key Medical Center Announce New Program for Pregnant Addicts," Sept. 18, 1990.

13 Lee Kennedy "New Center Serves Addicted Mothers, Addicted Babies," *Keynotes* 5(1), Winter 1990-91, 10-11.

14 Press release, "CAP Program Results: Fewer NICU Births and Significant Savings," Jan. 15, 1992; "CAP Program Shows Positive Results After One Year," June 19, 1992.

15 Press release, Oct. 10, 1990 on Waters; press release, Oct. 12, 1990 on Gregerman.

16 Press release, "Bush Names Key Volunteers 457th 'Daily Point of Light,'" May 16, 1991.

17 Press release, "Francis Scott Key Medical Center Dedicates $17 Million Geriatrics Center on Bayview Campus," June 2, 1991.

18 *Ibid.*

19 "Aged to Perfection," *Bayviews* 7(1), Winter 1994, 24-25.

20 Transcript of videotape of dedication ceremony of Johns Hopkins Geriatrics Center, June 6, 1991.

21 *Ibid.*

22 Transcript of videotape of groundbreaking for acute care patient tower, Oct. 15, 1991; press release, "Francis Scott Key Medical Center Announces New Name for Facility," Jan. 31, 1994, with accompanying fact sheet.

23 Transcript of Peterson speech at dedication of Francis Scott Key Pavilion, April 26-27, 1994.

24 Transcript of Harvey speech at ground-breaking for Francis Scott Key Pavilion, Oct. 15, 1991.

25 Press release, "The Francis Scott Key Medical Center Celebrates Groundbreaking of New Hospital Tower," Oct. 4, 1991; transcript of videotape of groundbreaking ceremony, Oct. 15, 1991.

26 *Ibid.*, transcript of 10/15/91 groundbreaking ceremony video.

27 *Ibid.*

28 *Community News* 2(2), Fall 1990, 5.

29 *Ibid.*

30 Jennifer Lamb-Korn, "Coming of Age at the Johns Hopkins Geriatrics Center," *Community News* 3(1), Spring 1991, 2-3.

31 *Ibid.*

32 *Ibid.*, 3.

33 Sandy Reckert-Reusing, "Spirit of Giving," *Community News* 6(1), Fall 1993, 1-2.

34 Press release, "Post Acute AIDS Unit Opens at FSKMC," July 29, 1992.

35 *Ibid.*; Lisa DeNike, "A New Focus on Patient Care," *Keynotes* 6(1), Spring 1993, 12-13.

36 Press release, July 29, 1992.

37 Kim Goad, "Defining Quality Service: People Power," *Keynotes* 6(1), Spring 1993, 6-9.

38 *Ibid.*

39 Slides in 2001 Bayview Medical Center presentation.

40 "Trend of Excess of Revenue Over Expenses," fiscal years 1985-1995, list from Grabill.

41 Press release, "First Stone Center in State Opens at Francis Scott Key Medical Center," Jan. 3, 1994.

42 *Ibid.*

43 *Ibid.*

44 *Bayviews* 7(1), Winter 1994, "AESOP," Sandy Reckert-Reusing, *Keynotes* 6(1), Spring 1993, 6.

45 *Ibid.*, 7.

46 *Ibid.*

47 Grabill int. 10/1/03.

48 *Ibid.*

49 *Ibid.*

50 Press release, "Francis Scott Key Medical Center Announces New Name for Facility," Jan. 31, 1994; transcript of video of FSK Pavilion dedication, Apr. 26-27, 1994; Peterson speech, 4/26/94.

51 Transcript of video of FSK Pavilion dedication, 4/26/94.

52 *Community News* 5(1), Spring 1994, back page.

53 Press release, Oct. 4, 1991, on groundbreaking for "$61 million, 190-bed" acute patient care tower.

54 Peterson speech at dedication, Apr. 26, 1994.

55 "Building Our Future," *Keynotes* 6(1), Spring 1993, 24; Peterson speech at dedication, Apr. 26, 1994; "Aged to Perfection," *Bayviews* 7(1), Spring 1994, 24; *Community News* 5(1), Spring 1994, "A Quick Glance..." (description of Key Pavilion)

56 Transcript of FSK Pavilion dedication ceremony, Apr. 26-27, 1994.

57 *Ibid.*

58 *Ibid.*

59 *Bayview News*, 6(3), Spring 1995, 8.

60 Block letter to "Hopkins Family Member," May 25, 1995.

61 *Ibid.*

62 Peterson letter to Bayview employees, May 25, 1995.

63 Ward int.

64 Press release, "Roxbury Native Named President and CEO of Johns Hopkins Bayview Medical Center," Sept. 1, 1999; press release "Gregory F. Schaffer Named Vice President of Support Services at Johns Hopkins Bayview Medical Center," Aug. 21, 1995.

65 Press releases, May 4, 1995 (Munster) and Nov. 14, 1995 (Schuster).

66 Bayview PowerPoint presentation, 2001.

67 Memo from Ken Grabill, Oct. 1, 2003, with accompanying list of "Trend of Excess Revenue over Expenses, Fiscal Years 1985-1995."

68 Peterson int. 7/21/03.

Chapter Five

1 John Fairhall, *The Sun*, "Hopkins system fills No. 2 slot," May 27, 1995.

2 *Ibid.*

3 Kastor, John A., M.D. *Governance of Teaching Hospitals: Turmoil at Penn and Hopkins* (Baltimore: Johns Hopkins University Press, 2003), 213-277.

4 *Ibid.*, 224-226.

5 *Ibid.*, 230.

6 *Ibid.*, 232.

7 *Ibid.*, 232-236.

8 Peterson e-mail to author, March 3, 2004; "Judy Reitz Appointed Executive Vice President and Chief Operating Officer of the Johns Hopkins Hospital," press release, Oct. 12, 1999.

9 Media Advisory, "Johns Hopkins Bayview ... Breaks Ground on a New Ambulatory Care Center," April 29, 1996; press release, "Johns Hopkins Bayview Medical Center Dedicates New Outpatient Facility," May 17, 1999.

10 Press release, "Johns Hopkins Bayview Opens First of Its Kind Motility and Digestive Disorders Center," Nov. 18, 1996; attachments on Marvin M. Schuster, M.D.; "What Are Motility Disorders?"; "Motility Disorders Affect Millions Both Physically and Financially."

11 *Ibid.*

12 *Ibid.*

13 Press release, "Blaustein Foundation Supports Schuster Center at Hopkins Bayview," May 23, 1997.

14 *Bayview News* 6(3), Spring 1995, 4.

15 *Bayview News* Winter 1997, 6; *Bayview News* 11(1) Winter 1998, 3.

16 Sandy Reckert-Reusing, "The Gift of a Lifetime," *Bayview News* 9(1) Spring 1996, 2; Janet Farrar Worthington, "Overweight? The Problem May Be A Faulty Gene," *Bayview News* 9(1) Spring 1996, 1; 8.

17 *Ibid.*

18 *Bayview News* 11(3), Fall 1998, 5; *Bayview News*, 16(1) Sandy Reckert-Reusing, "Mini Hip," 3; press release, "Drs. James & Lidia Wenz Killed In Accident," Jan. 20 , 2004.

19 *Bayview News* 11(3), Fall 1998, 5

20 Kim Goad, "On the Cutting Edge," *Bayview News* 11(2), Spring 1998, 1; 8.

21 Janet Farrar Worthington, "Overweight? The Problem May Be A Faulty Gene," *Bayview News* 9(1) Spring 1996, 1; 8.

22 *Ibid.*

23 Kim Goad, "The Results Are In! Community assessment project paints a health-related picture of the neighborhoods we serve," *Bayview News* 10(3), Fall 1997, 6; interview with Gregory Schaffer, Dec. 9, 2003 (hereinafter "Schaffer int.").

24 Schaffer int.

25 Schaffer int., Sandy Reckert-Reusing, "Mothering Comes Naturally To Us," *Bayview News* 10(3), Fall 1997, 1.

26 *Bayview News* 10(2), "Hopkins Bayview Online," 2

27 "Expanding to Bring Hopkins-Quality Care to You," *Bayview News* 11(3), Fall 1998, 2.

28 *Bayview News* 14(1) Summer 1999, "Bayview Community Practices," 3.

29 *Bayview News*, Vol. 11, No. 3 Fall 1998, 7.

30 Media advisory, "Innovative Hopkins Elder Plus Program Demonstrates Why Future of Long-term Care Depends Less on Nursing Homes," Jan. 9, 1997.

31 *Ibid.*

32 Mary Ann Ayd, "Health on Wheels: Bayview maps a new route to neighborhood care," *Bayview News* 15(2), Fall 2000, 1; 7.

33 Kim Goad, "Brain Power," *Bayview News* 10(1), Winter 1997, 1; 7.

34 *Ibid.*, Kim Goad "Bayview Goes Global," 3.

35 Sandy Reckert-Reusing, "An Element of Danger," *Bayview News* 11(1), Winter 1998, 5.

36 Kim Goad, "FX to RX," *Bayview News* 13(1), Spring 1999, 3; Robert Spence e-mail to author, April 3, 2004.

37 "Bayview's Top Docs," *Bayview News* 11(1), Winter 1998, 7.

38 Press release, "Trustees Announce Leadership Changes at Johns Hopkins Bayview Medical Center," Aug. 30, 1999.

39 "Leadership Changes at Hopkins Bayview" and "JHBP Introduces Its New President," *Bayview News*, Fall 1999.

40 Schaffer int.

Chapter Six

1 Kim Goad, "Beating the Clock: Hopkins Bayview Prepares for Y2K," *Bayview News* 14(1), Summer 1999, 3.

2 *Ibid.*

3 Kim Goad, "In an Emergency, You Can Count on Bayview," *Bayview News* 15(1), Summer 2000, 3.

4 *Ibid.*

5 "Making Emergency 'Room': Johns Hopkins Bayview Emergency Department Expansion," *Bayview News* 15(3), Winter 2001, 8; Adams int., 3/31/04.

6 Press release, "David Hellmann Joins Hopkins Bayview as Chairman of the Department of Medicine," Aug. 28, 2000.

7 Interviews with Chester Schmidt; Burton D'Lugoff; Philip Zieve; Gregory Schaffer; T-shirt owned by Robert D. Chessin, M.D., Hopkins School of Medicine, 1972.

8 Author's interview with Robert D.H. Harvey, Apr. 5, 2004 (hereinafter "Harvey int.").

9 D'Lugoff int.

10 Schmidt int.

11 Schaffer int.

12 *Ibid.*

13 Schaffer int.

14 Kastor, *Governance of Teaching Hospitals*, 183.

15 "Hopkins Merges Faculty Groups," *Bayview News* 16(3), Winter 2002, 8.

16 *Ibid.*; Kastor, *Governance of Teaching Hospitals*, 183-184 and fn. 92, 337.

17 Dean's Letter, 2/8/01, from Edward Miller to colleagues.

18 Schaffer int.

19 Johns Hopkins Bayview Medical Center FY '03 Accomplishments, 1; press release, "Hopkins Bayview Named to '100 Top Hospitals': ICU Benchmarks for Success," Feb. 13, 2001.

20 "Bayview Opens Doors to New Vascular Center" *Bayview News* 15(2), Fall 2000, 8.

21 "The Wait is Over," *Bayview News* 16(1), Summer 2001, 3; "Clinics on the Move," *Bayview News* 15(3), Winter 2001, 4.

22 "Rehabilitation Department Undergoes Rehab," *Bayview News* 16(2), Fall 2001, 8; Cassie Gainer, "Renovation, Transformation, Rehabilitation," *Bayview News* 17(2) Fall 2002, 6-7.

23 Media advisory, "Special Invitation to Reporters and Producers: Experience First Hand the Future of Orthopedics," 9/16/02; Sandy Reckert-Reusing, "Presenting the Future of Orthopaedics: Bayview opens International Center for Orthopaedic Advancement," *Bayview News* 17(3), Winter 2003, 4.

24 Cassie Gainer, "Ready, Set ... PET," *Bayview News* 16(1), Summer 2001, 1; 7.

25 *Ibid.*

26 *Ibid.*

27 Sandy Reckert-Reusing, "Doctoring Hospitals: Hospitalist movement delivers more efficient, better outcome health care," *Bayview News* 16(2), Fall 2001, 3.

28 Sandy Reckert-Reusing, "Children's Medical Practice: Big on 'Little' Experience," *Bayview News* 16(3), Winter 2002, 1; 7.

29 Kim Goad, "Update on Aging," *Bayview News* 17(2), Fall 2002, 3; press release, "Study Finds Relationship Between Geriatric Frailty, Biology," Nov. 15, 2002.

30 Press release, "Study Finds Relationship Between Geriatric Frailty, Biology," Nov. 15, 2002.

31 Kim Goad, "Bayview Physicians Makes a Sound Investment in Dundalk," *Bayview News* 14(2) Fall 1999, 4; Kim Goad, "Movin' on Up: Closing of Northpoint Medical Center routes patients to JHBP's new & improved facilities," *Bayview News* 14(3), Winter 2000, 4; "Building a Better Health Center," *Bayview News* 14(4), Spring 2000, 7.

32 Kim Goad, "Hopkins Expands Its Reach," *Bayview News* 15(1), Summer 2000, 7; press release, "Johns Hopkins Dedicates New Center at White Marsh," Sept. 20, 2000.

33 Press release, "Hopkins ElderPlus Granted Permanent PACE Status," Aug. 23, 2002; Schaffer int.

34 Johns Hopkins Bayview Medical Center FY '03 Accomplishments, 5; Lindsay Roylance, "Se Habla Espanol?" *Dome* 55(3), April 2004, 2.

35 Kim Goad, "Community Benefit Report," *Bayview News* 16(4), Spring 2002, special insert.

36 *Ibid.*

37 Sandy Reckert-Reusing, "Diving Into His Work: Bayview Surgeon Gets His Feet Wet at the Aquarium," *Bayview News* 14(3), Winter 2000, 1-2.

38 P. Susan Davis, "Book Review: A Face First," *Bayview News* 16(2) Fall 2001, 7.

39 Press release, "The Johns Hopkins Geriatric Center Building Renamed to Honor John R. Burton, M.D.," May 30, 2003; Dani Mardayat, "It's All in the Name," *Bayview News* 18(1) Summer 2003, 8.

40 Press release, "Bayview Announces New Name for Geriatrics Center," Oct. 15, 2003.

41 "Bayview's 'Top Docs'," *Bayview News* 17(3), Winter 2003, 7.

42 Press release, "Bayview Appoints New Clinical Research Director," Apr. 18, 2002; Johns Hopkins Bayview Medical Center FY '03 Accomplishments, 28.

43 "Congratulations Bayview News!" *Bayview News* 14(4), Spring 2000, 8.

44 Press release, "Hopkins Bayview Names Vice President of Medical Affairs," Jan. 28, 2003.

45 "New VP of Medical Affairs," *Bayview News* 18(2), Fall 2003, 4.

46 Johns Hopkins Bayview Medical Center FY '03 Accomplishments, 2.

47 *Ibid.*

48 E-mail from Carl Francioli on Bayview growth and financial figures, Apr. 6, 2004.

49 Johns Hopkins Bayview Medical Center FY '03 Accomplishments, 8; e-mail from Carl Francioli, Apr.6, 2004.

50 Harvey int.

51 Jim Duffy, "Greg Schaffer on Bayview's Bright Future," *Dome*, 55(3), Spring 2004, 7.

52 *Ibid.*

53 *Ibid.*; Schaffer int.

54 "Putting the Past Behind: Bayview Physicians and Their East Baltimore Colleagues Are Sharing Center Stage Since Their Merger," *Change* 7(3), Feb. 14, 2003, 3.

55 *Ibid.*

56 "Putting the Past Behind," *Change*, 7(3), Feb. 14, 2003, 3; *Dome*, 55(3), Spring 2004, 7; Reitz int.

57 Reitz int.

58 Peterson e-mail to author, Mar. 22, 2004.

59 *Ibid.*

60 Zieve int. 12/17/03.

61 *Ibid.*

CHRONOLOGY

1773
The Maryland General Assembly authorizes the purchase of 20 acres outside the northwest border of Baltimore city as the site for the Baltimore City and County Almshouse, which opened in 1774. The land cost 350 pounds of tobacco, then a common currency.

1789-1801
Andrew Wiesenthal (1762-1798), an accomplished diagnostician, and James Smith (1771-1841), a student of the renowned Benjamin Rush of Philadelphia, serve as attending physicians at the Baltimore Almshouse. Wiesenthal also offers medical instruction at another Baltimore location for a class of 15 students (1789-90). Smith performs Maryland's first vaccination for smallpox at the Almshouse on May 1, 1801. He becomes known as "the Jenner of America" for his advocacy of vaccination.

1812
William Gibson and Samuel Baker of the College of Medicine of Maryland (later the University of Maryland Medical School) accept appointments as visiting physicians and use the residents of the Almshouse as subjects for medical instruction.

1822
The Almshouse moves to Calverton, once the estate of a city merchant, on 306 acres in the then-rural area now bordered by Franklin, Presstman, Lexington and Pulaski streets. By outward appearances an impressive structure, the Almshouse at Calverton actually was built on swampland. Its water supply was vulnerable to raw sewage, and its land was a fertile breeding ground for disease-carrying mosquitoes.

1840
William Power (1813-1852), a Yale and University of Maryland graduate, becomes resident physician at Calverton and begins the practice of scientific medicine in Baltimore, introducing careful medical histories and post-mortem examinations.

1866
Residents of Calverton are moved to a new 240-acre site far outside the Baltimore city limits, into a new $500,000, three-story building on an eastern crest overlooking the Chesapeake Bay. Named the "Baltimore Bay View Asylum" to reflect the institution's role as an insane asylum, as well as a place for the poor and those needing medical care, the original three-story building has since evolved into today's Mason F. Lord Building.

1871
The first paying patients are admitted to the Bay View Asylum.

1885
The plight of the insane residents of Bay View is among the factors that bring the facility to the attention of William H. Welch (1850-1934), the famed first professor of pathology at the new Johns Hopkins School of Medicine, beginning the association between Hopkins and its future Eastern Avenue sibling that has lasted 120 years. Welch's assistant, William Thomas Councilman (1854-1933), a pathologist at Bay View since 1879 and later a renowned professor of pathology at Harvard Medical School, and other Hopkins physicians become visitors at Bay View.

1886
Hopkins begins staffing Bay View's hospital for the insane.

1890
Bay View establishes separate wards for the treatment of patients with pulmonary tuberculosis; these are probably the first separate tuberculosis wards in any general hospital in the United States.

1890s
Hopkins' development of a system of student and residency training is adopted at Bay View, and Hopkins medical students begin examining a wide range of patients there. Hopkins, the University of Maryland Medical School and the College of Physicians and Surgeons (now Mercy Hospital) nominate residents, assistant residents and medical students to the city-appointed trustees of Bay View for assignment there.

1911
Thomas R. Boggs, a protégé of Sir William Osler and an associate professor of medicine at Johns Hopkins, is named chief of medicine and Arthur M. Shipley, superintendent of the University of Maryland Hospital, is named surgeon in chief at Bay View. Both men would guide the institution for the next 27 years. (Boggs became president of the Association of American Physicians in 1937.)

1911
A new, state-of-the-art hospital building for the medical and surgical wards and a nurses' training school open at Bay View.

1923
Colonel (later Brigadier General) Rufus E. Longan, former executive officer of the Port of New York during World War I, is appointed the first professional superintendent of Bay View.

1925
Bay View Asylum is renamed Baltimore City Hospitals. The plural "s" reflects the fact that multiple hospitals exist on the same site to deliver acute care, chronic care and care of tuberculosis patients.

1929
At the urging of both The Johns Hopkins University and the University of Maryland, Baltimore city completes plans to erect a $2.75 million new general hospital, tuberculosis

sanitarium, service building and nurses' home at City Hospitals. Winford Smith, director of the Johns Hopkins Hospital, serves as architectural consultant.

1931-37
A new nurses' home opens in 1931; a 450-bed general hospital (the present A Building) opens in 1935, along with the north section of the B Building. In 1935, City Hospitals is placed under the control of the new Baltimore City Department of Public Welfare. A new tuberculosis sanitarium opens in 1937.

1930
Alan Chesney, dean of the Johns Hopkins School of Medicine, an important ally of the City Hospitals administration, works with colleagues at the University of Maryland medical school to enhance the relationship between City Hospitals and the medical schools. City Hospitals staff physicians are appointed to the faculties of both medical schools, and patients at City Hospitals continue to be used in teaching the universities' medical students.

1940
The U.S. Public Health Service establishes a research unit of the new Department of Gerontology, under Edward J. Stieglitz.

1941
Nathan Shock joins Stieglitz's department and begins developing programs in gerontology that would become world-famous.

1945
Lingering personnel problems prompted by World War II staffing shortages lead to creation of first full-time positions of chiefs of the pediatrics, X-ray and pathology departments.

1948
Baltimore city voters approve an $8 million bond issue to improve City Hospitals, including renovation of the acute care hospital and construction of a new tuberculosis unit.

1954
Harold Harrison publishes research on preventing diarrhea in babies through oral rehydration therapy, hailed by the British medical journal The Lancet as "potentially the most important medical advance this century."

1955
City Hospitals' surgery unit ends a 45-year tradition by opposing the appointment of the

University of Maryland's nominee as surgeon in chief and urges the appointment of Mark M. Ravitch, a highly regarded Hopkins-trained surgeon. The University of Maryland, resentful of this move, begins its gradual withdrawal from association with City Hospitals. (Later, Thomas Turner, dean of the Hopkins School of Medicine, establishes agreement with the University of Maryland's school of medicine under which City Hospitals would become a teaching venue exclusively for Johns Hopkins medical students, and the University of Maryland's medical students would be taught at a Veterans Administration hospital built next to the University of Maryland in Baltimore.)

1958
Peter Safar, the first full-time chief of anesthesiology at City Hospitals, pioneers mouth-to-mouth resuscitation and creates City Hospitals' medical-surgical multidisciplinary intensive care unit; it is first ICU in the country with 24-hour coverage by anesthesiologists. Nathan Shock and Reuben Andres begins the Baltimore Longitudinal Study in City Hospitals' Gerontology Research Center's Clinical Physiology Branch.

1960
City Hospitals physicians receive many honors. Harold Harrison receives gold medal from the American Academy of Pediatrics and its $1,000 Borden Prize; Nathan Shock, now chief of research in gerontology, is chosen by Modern Medicine as one of the 10 outstanding biological scientists of 1960; Mark M. Ravitch, chief of the Department of Surgery, becomes editor of both Surgery magazine and The Quarterly Review of Surgery; Francis Chinard, head of the Department of Medicine, is elected to New York Academy of Sciences and serves as editor of The American Journal of Physiology and the Journal of Applied Physiology.

1962
City Hospitals' cancer chemotherapy unit, begun by Albert Owens with a few beds in the Tuberculosis Hospital, is moved to the B Building with a complete staff and laboratory equipment. It will provide the foundation for oncology research and treatment at The Johns Hopkins Hospital.

1963
The new City Hospitals Department of Chronic and Community Medicine is created under the direction of Mason F. Lord, whose innovative concepts for applying principles of preventive medicine to the treatment of elderly people would become prototypes for similar systems nationwide.

1965
City Hospitals is separated from Baltimore's Department of Welfare and becomes the operation of a new city Department of Hospitals.

1968
The Kiwanis Burn Unit, later the Baltimore Regional Burn Center, opens with the aid of $20,000 raised by the Kiwanis Club of Highlandtown. Over the next 30 years, the club, known now as the Kiwanis Club of East Baltimore, would donate more than $1 million to the burn center, which has treated thousands of burn patients from the Mid-Atlantic region.

The National Institute on Aging, one of the U.S. government's National Institutes of Health, completes its new $7.5 million, four-story Gerontology Research Center at City Hospitals.

1972
Physicians at City Hospitals create Chesapeake Physicians, P.A. (Professional Association), a unique faculty practice plan, which immediately increases the budget for physicians and other medical staff.

1973
City Hospitals celebrates its bicentennial and proudly cites its accomplishments in the shadow of growing financial problems. Its annual deficit is nearly $6 million.

1975
City Hospitals is said to have a projected deficit of $8.5 million.

1976
Most of City Hospitals' financial leadership is dismissed by Mayor William Donald Schaefer; day-to-day management is assumed by the city's Department of Finance, headed by Charles L. Benton Jr.

1980
City voters approve a charter amendment to transform City Hospitals into a public-interest corporation, called The Medical Center of Baltimore, Inc. Mayor Schaefer tries unsuccessfully to persuade the state to assume control of City Hospitals, then begins exploring bids from for-profit health care companies to take over its operation.

1981
Robert Heyssel, then executive vice president and soon to be president of The Johns Hopkins Hospital, discusses with Edward Halle, Hopkins

Hospital's senior vice president for administration, the need for Hopkins to determine if it wants to bid to manage City Hospitals. Hopkins begins a feasibility study to assess this option.

1982
Mayor Schaefer announces that he has suggested Hopkins, rather than a for-profit health care company, assume management of City Hospitals on behalf of the city. Heyssel and Richard Ross, dean of the Hopkins School of Medicine, decide that if Hopkins could start reducing City Hospitals' staggering deficits during a trial management period, perhaps Hopkins should consider taking it over. The Hopkins Hospital board of trustees approves initiation of formal negotiations for acquiring City Hospitals. In August, the Baltimore City Board of Estimates approves the City Hospitals' management contract for the new Johns Hopkins Health Plan, a managed care company.

Ronald Peterson, administrator of Hopkins' Children's Medical and Surgical Center, becomes executive director of City Hospitals on September 13, 1982. He is joined by William Ward, former associate administrator of the Johns Hopkins Oncology Center, as chief operating officer and Kenneth Grabill, an associate director of operations, planning and budgets at Hopkins Hospital, as chief financial officer.

1983
The leadership team of Peterson, Ward and Grabill dramatically reduces City Hospitals' deficits, wiping nearly $7 million in red ink off the books in less than a year. In February, Peterson reports to Hopkins' joint committee of trustees detailing the financial turnaround at City Hospitals and recommending that Hopkins acquire it. Later, the joint board unanimously approves initiation of formal negotiations for the takeover of City Hospitals.

1984
Hopkins and the city conclude negotiations in March, providing for the transfer of City Hospitals' ownership to Hopkins on July 1. The parties agree that if Hopkins cannot operate City Hospitals successfully after five years, the university can return it to the city. In a formal transfer ceremony on July 2, Hopkins takes over City Hospitals, renames it the Francis Scott Key Medical Center and names Peterson its president.

1985
Hopkins reduces the Francis Scott Key Medical Center's deficit to just $500,000; by the end of fiscal 1986, FSKMC is in the black, recording a $2.6

million "excess of revenues over expenses." It has remained in the black ever since. Master planning begins in June, the same month the National Institute on Drug Abuse opens its renovated Addiction Research Center.

1986
The Johns Hopkins Healthcare System (JHHS) is created, including The Johns Hopkins Hospital, the Francis Scott Key Medical Center and three other health care providers then associated with Hopkins. FSKMC is a major contributor to JHHS's vitality and growth.

1988
Groundbreaking is held for Phase I of the FSKMC redevelopment program, the centerpiece of which will be the $15.5 million, 130,000-square-foot geriatrics center.

1989
The Johns Hopkins School of Medicine opens its Asthma & Allergy Center at FSKMC.

1991
The Johns Hopkins Geriatrics Center opens, completing Phase I of FSKMC redevelopment program. Ground is broken for Phase II of FSKCM redevelopment program, the centerpiece of which will be the $63 million, 275,000-square-foot acute care tower.

1993
FSKMC's profits rise 85 percent to $3.7 million on revenues of $157 million; occupancy of 73 percent is better than the statewide average.

1994
FSKMC is renamed the Johns Hopkins Bayview Medical Center. The new acute care tower, the Francis Scott Key Pavilion, opens.

1996
Peterson becomes president of The Johns Hopkins Hospital and remains president of Bayview. Ground is broken for a $13 million, 98,000-square-foot ambulatory care center and medical offices.

1999
Gregory Schaffer succeeds Peterson as president of Bayview Medical Center. Bayview Medical Offices and outpatient facility open.

2000
David Hellmann, executive vice chairman and residency program director for the Department of Medicine at The Johns Hopkins Hospital, moves

to Hopkins Bayview to become the new chairman of its department of medicine, succeeding Philip Zieve.

2001
Phase II of Bayview Medical Offices building is completed.

Johns Hopkins School of Medicine names L. Reuven Pasternak its first vice dean for Bayview.

2002
Johns Hopkins Bayview Physicians (formerly Chesapeake Physicians) faculty practice group merges with Johns Hopkins' Clinical Practice Association (CPA), uniting the faculty practices of both hospitals under the CPA.

2003
U.S. News & World Report magazine names Johns Hopkins Geriatrics, based at Hopkins Bayview, the number one program of its kind in the nation. In *Baltimore* magazine's annual survey of the region's "Top Docs," 13 physicians at Hopkins Bayview are cited as the best in their fields.

Johns Hopkins Bayview reports growth in every facet of its operations except the average patient's length of stay, which declines slightly.

Richard D. Bennett succeeds Philip Zieve as Hopkins Bayview's vice president for medical affairs.

Linda Fried is appointed director of the Division of Geriatric Medicine and Gerontology, succeeding John R. Burton. *The Daily Record* newspaper names Fried one of Maryland's "Top 100 Women for 2003."

The Hopkins Bayview geriatrics building is named the John R. Burton Pavilion, honoring Burton's leadership of the geriatrics program. The Geriatrics Center, located in the Burton Pavilion, itself is renamed the Johns Hopkins Bayview Care Center, reflecting the broad expansion of its services beyond nursing home care.

2004
The National Institutes of Health plans to erect a mammoth, 550,000-square-foot building for several of its existing programs on the campus, including the National Institute of Drug Abuse and National Institute on Aging's Gerontology Research Center.

INDEX

Page numbers shown in italic indicate illustrations.